The Cry in the Night

in the

Night

Dramas From the Life of a Doctor

Charles S Norburn, MD

Edited by Lillian Norburn Alexander

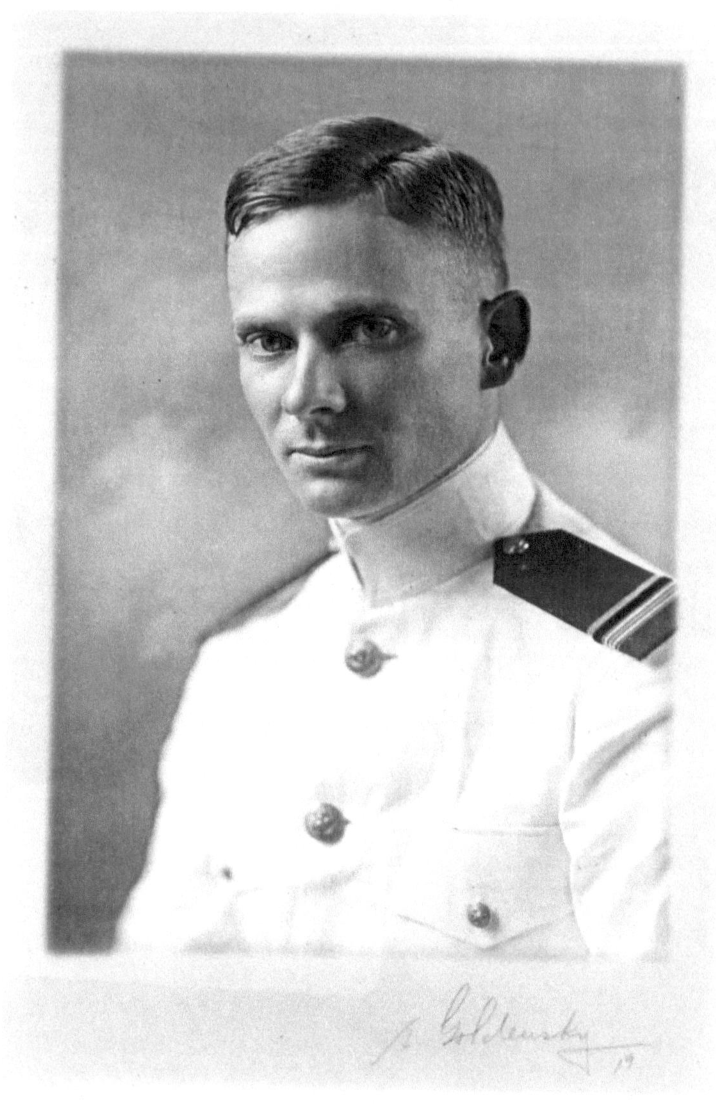

Elias Goldensky, "Charles S Norburn," Photograph. Photo courtesy of the collection of Lillian N Alexander.

First Edition

Charles S Norburn drew his inspiration from real life as do many authors. These stories are composites of situations and people from his experiences written as creative non-fiction.

Previous Publications:
Norburn, Charles S and Russell L Norburn. *Mankind's Greatest Step: A New Monetary System*. Vantage Press, Inc., 1971
Norburn, Charles S. *Throw Off the Yoke*. Omni Publications, 1979
Norburn, Charles S. *Honest Government: A Return to the U.S. Constitution*. New Puritan Library, 1984

ISBN: 979-8-21-805257-7

All photos courtesy of the Norburn family unless otherwise stated.

Cover design by Bruce Hester.

www.charlessnorburn.com

Contents

Preface

Many and varied interests filled the long life of Dr. Charles S Norburn. Born in 1890 in Thomasville, North Carolina, he witnessed vast changes in the world before his death at the age of 100. After attending the University of North Carolina and graduating early from the University of Virginia Medical School, he joined the Navy and served as a surgeon in WWI on hospital and transport ships.

In the 1920s, he moved to Asheville, North Carolina and started a small, private hospital with his brother, Dr. Russell L Norburn. When the Norburn Hospital & Clinic outgrew its facilities on Montford Avenue, it was moved to the former Normal School property on Biltmore Avenue. The hospital now utilized the Normal School's large 32-acre campus with its dormitory, library, and laundry. The scale of Dr. Norburn's vision for this property as a major medical complex was only partially realized under his direction before its merger in 1950 with Victoria Hospital. In the ensuing years, his dream of a large hospital there, serving the region, has come to fruition.

He loved life, the wonder and beauty of nature, and had a delightful sense of humor. A true Renaissance man, he was well versed in music, literature, antiques, history, philosophy, architecture, and mathematics among other things. His collections included paintings, antiques, and pipe organs. He acquired several patents that became standard on every organ manufactured. He collected fine woodworking and blacksmith tools and was a craftsman himself creating many finely carved furnishings. Owning and managing a small dairy farm occupied his spare time for some years and then the restoration of an 18th century beach house on Pawleys Island, South Carolina.

His love of literature led him to write even as a young boy. He wrote of his medical training, his time in the Navy, and his medical career. He published several books on the US monetary system when he was in his 80s and 90s.

The main characters of these dramas in this book are his patients with whom he felt deep empathy. He wrote of their lives and deaths and their struggles with the vicissitudes of life. Included are episodes not only of the gruesome realities in the life of a doctor but also the gratifying.

The book is filled with his spirit, his thoughts on the human condition, the medicine of his time, and his devotion to the people and places of his long medical career.

Many people have helped in the publication of this book. A special thanks to Susan Oleaga and Jeff Dodge for research, Debra Cooper for excellent editing and proofreading, Lauren Harr of Gold Leaf Literary for her publishing expertise, and especially to Diana Corbin for her encouragement, collaboration, and invaluable copywriting and editing skills without which the project could not have been done.

This book is dedicated to all those whose lives were touched by Charles S Norburn and is a small tribute to this extraordinary man who was my father.

Lillian Norburn Alexander

As if in Prologue

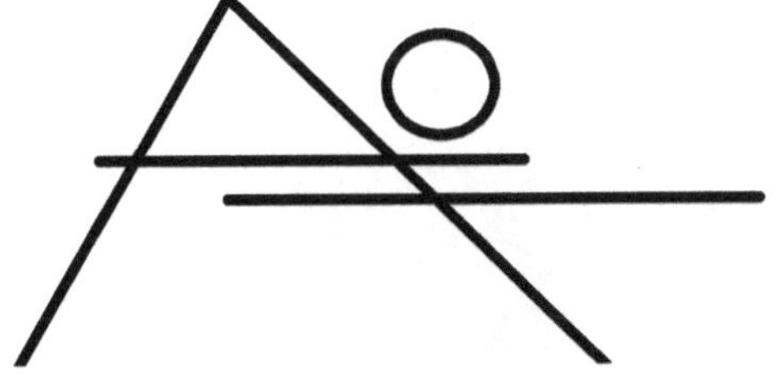

As if in Prologue

These dramas have been selected from among those that occurred during my long years of practice. Since their portrayal is colored—perhaps even more than is usually the case—by the observer's personality, his experience, and his sympathy. It may not be amiss to tell briefly what these have been.

The surgical handling of my patients was all in the day's work, done and soon forgotten. This labor was but a means to an end—that of restoring my patients to health. It was the human, the personal, side of medicine that left upon me its lasting impressions. For always as I worked, there was the consciousness of the transcendent value of the individual's life, of the devotion and interdependence that exist between a patient and his family, of the finality of failure.

Looking back, I realize that I had the trait of high meditative and personal interest in human beings apart from their illnesses at the time I entered the hospital wards as a student. The only patients of those days whom I remember distinctly are those who moved me in this respect.

One of the first patients assigned to me was a young farmer. He was tall and rawboned and had long, thick, straw-colored hair. His wife told me they lived on a small, rented farm and they had two little children. In her face I could read a double anxiety. She was fearful not only for her husband but also for the safety of the breadwinner.

After taking the history and examining the patient, I made a diagnosis that was confirmed by the surgeon.

At sundown I followed my patient into the operating room to observe his operation. Though nothing was said, I could sense that it did not go well.

All night I awoke and thought and feared then slept and dreamed of him and woke again. At daybreak I put on my clothes and went, not to the ward, but to the morgue. A long form laid there, a tag tied to its toe. The face was hidden by a cloth wound about the head from which projected a shock of long, coarse, blond hair.

I failed to see the significant fact, the ironic twist, the new or unusual universal relationship that would have made this happening a drama in the sense of those recorded here. Perhaps, if I had talked again with the wife and had learned the patient's background, I might have seen what lay behind appearances and now would have another title to add to my list. Or perhaps the true and profound significance of the tragedy had not yet developed and would not develop for many years.

It was, however, with no such thoughts that I sought the wife that morning but she had gone. She had left in the black of night to return to her poor home, to tell the news to her little children, and to plan for a new and uncertain future.

These then are the forms I see when I look back—patients and their families acting under stress and reacting to it as they faced the changing fortunes of life while almost every conceivable emotion sweeps over them. I see these scenes and their relationships with the absolute and great moving forces of nature.

Many scenes that crowd through my memory are but fragmentary. Some, however, have all the elements of a drama, complete in groundwork and plot.

It may seem to the reader that I have selected too many stories of tragedy. He knows full well that in little more than the length of time covered by the events of this book the span of man's life has doubled; that medicine and surgery, in keeping with our rapidly changing world, have in that time also improved almost beyond belief; that save in terminal cases hospital stays have taken on an air of assurance, with a happy outcome all but routine. To this I shall say that these stories have been selected solely for their human interest. Tragedies such as these are forever with us, whether we shut our eyes to them or not.

Strange to most readers are the settings of some of the stories. The once-so-true description of an asylum is an example of this. Modern management and methods have changed this greatly. The types of cases treated are, however, the same. Another setting, remembered by the older generation but in our land seen no more, is the mill section of three-quarters of a century ago. Most of those who now work in the mills are in very different circumstances, they have little in common with the mill workers of earlier days. Yet, human nature itself has changed little and Nellie Morrison is still typical of those who are forced into environments foreign to their natures. Still so vivid in my mind is the picture of Nellie's last night that to me it seems as if she had lived her entire life for that one moment at its close. I tell the story almost as a sacred duty—to save such a heart from oblivion.

While attempting to portray the actors of these dramas, an old rule crossed my mind. It is that while verisimilitude is of great importance, a writer should not allow his readers to become too familiar with, too endeared to those characters marked for destruction. It has also been said that the storyteller should cushion the shock of an approaching tragedy by forecasting and preparing the reader for the blow. Fate, however, when it calls the turn, obeys no such rules. In life we know a person intimately. There are the thousands of remembered incidents, as well as our devotion and often love for those who are to die. In life, I say, we are not spared in this respect nor are we always prepared for an approaching tragedy—and here I write of life itself.

The vantage point that I have held has given me intimate knowledge of the players and their motives, made these stories possible and set them apart. The audience beyond the footlights may see these dramas only in part, may only partially understand their implications. I wish to take you with me into the wings backstage where you may hear the little asides, see the costumes, the make-up, as well as the stage itself.

The scenery is being shifted. The musicians are plucking the strings as they tune their instruments. Men and women are hurrying about. All are in truth actors, the real ones, making their last-minute preparations. They are oblivious of our presence, do not realize that it is a stage upon which they have wandered, and are unaware that their own names appear in the cast. The play will not be rehearsed. Even to those most concerned, its plot is still obscure. The players do not know what lines they are to speak. These are to be extemporaneous. The curtain lifts. The lights brighten. Soon now the drama is completed and makes way for another one to be played by other players amid other drops.

Here is a farce—much ado about nothing—but that also is life.

Here is what appears to be a puppet show, but here the puppets are men. Only we see the motives of those who pull the strings.

Now are played dramas in which terrible forms, unseen by the players but visible to us, stalk the stage amid the human beings or prompt them from the wings.

Now the scene is a railroad yard; now some barren, windswept waste.

A jester comes and shakes the bells upon his staff. The comedies are brief, their implications light. There is laughter. The players disperse, each to join another combination of actors upon another stage to play again, be the new play comedy or tragedy or those strange combinations of the two.

From our position in the wings, you will see that in the tragedies of life the weapons are real, whether they are held by fate itself or whether they are in the hands of the actors. The players who survive one drama in which others die will lose their own lives in the next in which they engage or, escaping that, the next.

The scenery shifts again. We shall see yet another drama in this never-ending series.

It is dark. The stars come out one by one. Dimly the stage is seen. This play is one of contemplation—of man's relations to those forces and those vast reaches forever beyond his ken. It seems to sum up all the rest.

This drama, too, now leads us through its several earlier acts. It is building to its climax. Every character, every force is becoming unified—aligned—now swiftly pointing, rushing to the end. The climax is reached, the thrust is made, the last line spoken, and all is silence.

There lies before us now—a nothingness—a vacant space. Still we sit, rapt for a moment, and gaze at the empty stage, the mind unable to throw off the spell cast over it.

There is no applause. Slowly now, we rise and move away, for here there is no curtain call.

The Bells

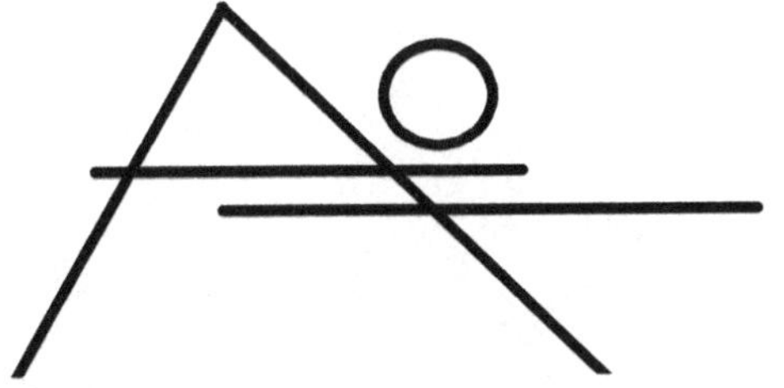

The Bells

As a second-year medical student, I held a minor position at the university infirmary and so, when the Christmas holidays came, did not go home but stayed with my work. One of my professors, Dr. Lawrence MacRae, was in charge of the infirmary. Sensing that I was homesick, he took me with him to see several of his private patients.

It was midafternoon on the day before Christmas when we turned onto Littleton Drive. The home was one of the older, more attractive homes of the village. I remarked on its well-kept and cheerful air and of the holly wreath on the door.

The patient, Howard Littleton, was in his early thirties, handsome and pleasant. He spoke to us with a voice of fine timbre but which carried a slight trembling and stammering. There was, too, a trembling of his hand as he held it out to me. To my inexperienced eye, he did not seem very ill.

"I am just nervous," he said. "I want something to make me sleep. Dolly would have me stay in bed."

The young wife, whom I knew to be the daughter of one of the professors, was statuesque and lovely—a fitting mate for the young man, I thought. On her countenance there seemed to be a slight cloud of disappointment and sadness, as well as of anxiety.

After we left her husband's room, she said, "Howard hasn't been himself since that little accident several days ago. He thought nothing of it but I wonder. He hasn't been able to sleep and when he has, there have been such strange dreams. He has been so restless since then."

As we left, I glanced through the door of another room and saw their little child and the lighted tree with its gaily wrapped packages beneath.

"Howard has been drinking too much lately," Dr. MacRae told me as we drove away. "It's an odd way to celebrate the holidays. He has delirium tremens."

Dr. MacRae supplemented my own knowledge of the young man and his family. Though his forebears had long been associated with the university as educators, Howard's father had gone into business and had accumulated, for that village and that time, a fortune. He had taken Howard, his only child, in as a partner and having taught him the business and its management, was now on the point of retiring.

"It seems to me," Dr. MacRae said, "that Howard by temperament was more suited to be an educator than he was to engage in business. He made a mistake."

In the gathering dusk we were back. As the wife met us in the hall, I knew from the look on her face that the hoped-for improvement had not taken place. Howard was much worse. He spoke to us, but his attention quickly strayed. With tremulous hands, he picked at the bedclothes. He was excited—turning, twisting, gazing tensely at spots on the wall—then suddenly shrinking back and crying out in fear.

The Bells

In an attempt to quiet him, more drugs were given. Also, arrangements were made for attendants and we drove away with Dr. MacRae's promise to return at nine o'clock.

Dr. MacRae was troubled and silent. He did not speak until he stopped his car to let me out. I thought perhaps he would say good-bye, but instead, he asked that I go with him to see Howard again that night.

When we returned, the Littleton household was thoroughly alarmed. Howard was sitting up in bed, trembling. His eyes were peering intently this way and that along the wall. They would fix upon some point; and then suddenly he would almost spring out of bed or else shrink back in terror, blurting out short sentences, pointing with a trembling finger to those fantastic images of his brain.

Friends sitting by the bed attempted to soothe him and when this failed, gently restrained him as the need arose.

Howard's elderly father—slender, tall, and straight—stood at the foot of the bed and looked down upon his son.

Nothing that Dr. MacRae did seemed to help. An hour went by and then another. Howard passed into an active and furious delirium. His face was congested; he was trembling, covered with sweat. He would stop his movements for a moment and stare, every muscle tensed to the breaking point, then spring in his frantic effort to escape. Now the walls were falling in upon him. Now all the machines at the mill were running backwards. Now horrible monsters raced through the vacant air.

Dr. MacRae had called in another physician. They were in consultation across the hall. They had tried many things without success. They had tried to hold him forcibly and anesthetize him but had finally given it up. In an attempt to control his rising temperature, cracked ice was placed upon him. He had thrown this off.

Howard was now a terrified wild animal struggling with its captors. Friends, acting in relays of four, exerted themselves to the utmost in an attempt to overcome his superhuman strength. If he ceased his struggle for a moment, merely speaking to him was enough to throw him into another wild convulsion.

In the midst of one of these violent outbursts, Howard suddenly ceased to struggle. He slumped back upon the bed. The men relaxed their grasp. He lay as if asleep with his eyes open. Puzzled and alarmed, I quickly stepped across the hall and asked Dr. MacRae to come. He took one look at Howard, turned to the dresser and, filling a hypodermic syringe with some drug, gave it to him. As Dr. MacRae filled the second syringe, I, whispering, asked him the trouble.

"He is dying," he said.

The news spread through the house. The friends who had been holding Howard faded from the room. The wife, in tears and sobbing prayer, fell upon her knees beside the bed.

"Don't take him from me, please—please!" she prayed.

The old father still stood erect at his place at the foot of the bed. He had not moved. The infant slept on in the adjoining room. Hopeless now, Dr. MacRae stood to one side.

I glanced at the dresser, littered with empty ampules, bottles, and syringes—all bearing mute testimony to man's pathetic helplessness when the tide of nature turns.

After a time, I said that if I could be of no aid I would go.

"Don't leave me now," the doctor said. Therefore, I stayed on and stood to one side as an observer to the course of this illness, of such a scene as I was destined to see again and again, and the events of this moment I was never to forget.

I could now see for myself that the changes in Howard were becoming more profound, that he was sinking deeper in his slumber, if such it might be called. His face became pallid. All expression faded. Slowly he sank. Dr. MacRae did those small things calculated to make him comfortable.

As the hour passed, Howard Littleton slowly settled lower and deeper and ever deeper and farther back. The pallor I had seen before had been only relative; it now became absolute.

Still the wife wept beside him and pled for his life. She poured out to him the story of their love, called attention to their child, spoke of her future loneliness.

Still the old father stood, straight and motionless, and gazed down at his son. His expression never changed. His eyes never wavered, never left the face before him. As if from some lofty vantage point, he saw the years of love and devotion, of pride and hope and expectation turn to dust and ashes.

The observers of this strange, eternal scene now stood rigid. That marvelous process we call life became ever weaker, fainter and then, almost imperceptible, flickered out at last.

Dr. MacRae leaned over and closed his patient's eyes.

There was a blurring of the outline of Howard's features, a remoteness about him, as if more than a breath separated him from the living.

The father never moved. The wife ceased her prayer and lowered her face to the bed.

A hush and an absolute stillness came to the room.

A moment later, a clear musical note broke in—the first of the now swelling, merry, joyous sound of bells. The wife and mother looked up.

"O God," she said, "It's Christmas."

Darkness

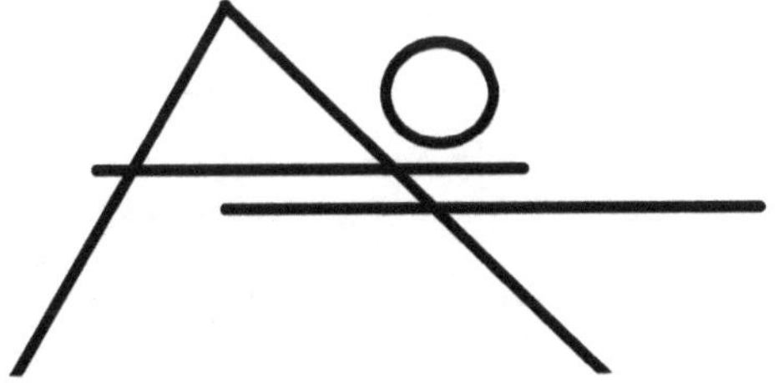

Darkness

The door of the small, unlighted, heavily shuttered house was cautiously opened and through the crack someone peered out into the gathering dusk. Slowly the door opened yet wider. A dark, slate-colored face appeared, and then a man's head was thrust out. He looked up into the sky and then to the right and to the left. A moment later he stepped out upon the stoop and closed the door. Pulling the wide brim of his black felt hat low over his eyes, he caught his turned-up collar, drew it high about his face, and came slowly down the steps. As he reached the sidewalk, he took another furtive glance about and then saw me sitting in my car. He stopped and with his dark hands still holding his coat collar close about his face, looked full at me.

My mission in that poor section of the city was to make a follow-up call on an accident case that had been discharged from the hospital the previous day. I had just driven up, stopped my car, and picked up my bag when my attention had been arrested by the slight sound and the movement as he opened his creaking door.

In depressed and thoughtful fascination I looked at the man, for I recognized at once that he was a victim of argyrism, a blackening of the skin caused by taking a preparation of silver.

The Cry in the Night

By a slow process of trial and error, doctors have, through the ages, advanced medicine step by step. Surely, few errors have been stranger and more heartbreaking than was one made a few years before I entered medical school. The professors there told me that the treatment of patients who suffered from gastric ulcers had always been unsatisfactory. After trying first one thing and then another, a chemical finally was found that bid fair to relieve this condition. It was a preparation of silver. The glad tidings spread and quite a number of patients were given the new treatment before its dreadful and irrevocable side effect became known. Those patients who had taken the silver preparation over a considerable period of time began to turn dark on the exposed surface of the body.

"It is nothing. It will clear up when the drug is stopped," some doctors said, but it didn't.

Those areas of the skin exposed to light continued to darken. The treatment was everywhere stopped, but for many the damage had already been done. It was found that the silver, uniting in the body with the chlorine of common table salt, had formed the white, insoluble compound of silver chloride. This compound, carried by the blood stream, was then deposited throughout the full thickness of the patient's skin; there was no way to remove this substance. It turned the skin into a living photographic film. When light struck these patients, their skin turned dark, just as light acts upon the silver compound in the usual photographic emulsion.

To stop the process, the patient must live forever in the darkness, yet few of those afflicted could do this. Careful as they might be, the process of darkening slowly and relentlessly continued. Every ray of light to which the patients were subjected made their color deeper. A few of these strangely afflicted people were still living in the great city where, as a postgraduate student, I worked. They lived mostly in seclusion although I had seen several of them. All were blighted and seared but none, it seemed to me, to such an extent as was the man before me. None had glanced into the sky with the same degree of intensity. None had looked at me with the same degree of bitterness as did he when, physician's bag in hand, I got out of the car and he recognized me as a doctor. I spoke to him, but he made no move and no sign that he heard. I turned from him and went in to make my call. After I finished the dressing, I inquired about the spectral figure I had just seen, but my patient could tell me little.

"I don't know his name," he said. He lives alone. He never comes out except at night."

The man with the slate-colored face and hands was gone when I returned to my car, but the images of what I had seen were not easily thrown off. It was hard to put from my mind the image of his tall, gaunt figure with the shoulders lifted and hunched forward and the black suit that hung almost in rags. Nor would I easily forget the powerful hands that clutched his coat collar and drew it up until it was only through a slit beneath his hat brim that his piercing eyes had looked so coldly into mine. Gradually over the next few days, under the press of work, these images finally slipped from my consciousness.

Yet a few more days passed and, in the middle of the night, I was awoken from a sound sleep by the ringing telephone.

"Doctor, this is Wade Barrett," said a strong, rather high-pitched voice. "I want you to make a call off Long Bridge Road. Just before you get to the bridge, there is a road leading to the left. Follow that road until you come to a high, woven fence, and then you will see the house."

"I don't practice medicine," I said. "I am a student and work in the charity wards."

"That is what I need," he said. "Other doctors won't come. Please come to see if I should go to the hospital."

"What is the matter?" I asked, and when he said he wanted me to decide that, I asked why he couldn't come to the clinic. He cut me short.

"You are a doctor, aren't you?" he asked, "and claim that you are one because you want to help people? Well, if anyone ever needed help I do now. Get dressed and come on."

There was something determined, something impelling in the voice. I heard the clatter of the telephone as he hung up the receiver. There didn't seem to be much choice; I got up and dressed. The way led through the slums of the city and on past the smoldering fires of garbage dumps. I then came upon a wide area in which there were no houses.

"Why in the world did I come?" I asked myself aloud as I left Long Bridge Road and saw the glow of the city far to my left. I was of half a mind to turn back. Now I came to the high fence and my lights showed the house beside the road. I stopped my car. There were no lights on in the house. It seemed more like a small office building than it did a residence. The broad gate in the fence was open. For a few moments I sat and looked about and wondered what to do.

There was some kind of sign on the building. I opened the car door and got out to read it. As I did so, I saw a tall form move in the shadow and a man stepped out. He was close beside me now and I could see that, though gaunt, he was of powerful physique. A long, heavy nightstick dangled by a thong from his right wrist, his hat was pulled low, and his left hand held his collar high about his face. I fell back, my heart jumped and began to race as I recognized the man to be the one who had looked at me with such ill will the week before.

"Turn off your lights—quick! Stop the motor," he commanded.

I had no weapon, not even a pocketknife. To oppose him would lead to a struggle which could have but one ending. I did as I was told. As I pushed in the light switch, all was plunged into darkness; and then, in the starlight, I saw him towering above me. He pointed with his nightstick. Together we passed through the gate. As he closed it, I heard its heavy lock snap shut.

"That path," he said. I entered the path and he followed.

It all seemed as unreal as a dream—a nightmare. It was hard to believe the man walking in my shoes was I.

How . . . why . . . how did I ever get here? I asked myself. He must have been given my name from that other patient.

There was a sharp chill to the night. The earth was soft and damp beneath my feet. The weeds that grew along the path were wet and as they struck against my clothes, cold water soaked through to the skin. This added to my nervous tension and caused my teeth to chatter. The air was heavy with the stench of hides and the musty odor of decay. As my eyes adjusted to the darkness, I saw that we were passing between piles of wrecked cars, old pipe, and other salvaged plunder of a large junkyard.

We came into the shadow of trees on a riverbank. I could see the dark water rippling past. Out of the darkness loomed a watchman's hut.

"Sit there," he ordered, pointing with his stick to a bench in the shadow by the door. He remained standing—also in shadow.

"You saw the house where I sleep," he said, suddenly breaking the silence. "Here is where I spend my waking hours. Once I was as fair as you are and life held just as much for me as it does for you. Now as a watchman in this cursed yard, I earn the bread that keeps my miserable life within me. You know why this has come about, don't you?"

"Yes," I answered simply.

"It is because I went to a doctor for aid. This is the way he gave it to me," he said, his voice becoming lower and more bitter.

"He was trying to help you," I broke in with some spirit. "This was a case of the best intentions going wrong. When a man has some disease for which there is no remedy, a doctor still must try to find one. Sometimes the new remedy works and sometimes it doesn't. If it relieves the patient, it will help men from then on. If it doesn't relieve him, the doctor has to try again. This mistake will never be repeated. Are you under the care of any doctor now?"

He made no reply. The silence dragged on.

"You asked me to come," I reminded him. "Are you sick?"

"Yes, I am sick," he said. "Sick unto death—sick of the cold, of the emptiness of life, of its loneliness!"

"Why don't you stay in the office and make your rounds from there?" I asked. "Why stay here away from everything that is human?"

"They are always burning lights there. This is the only place I fit—the only place I'm safe. I am a part of this wreckage," he replied.

A strange wistfulness had come into his voice. I began to feel surer of the outcome.

All at once he stiffened. "This is not what I brought you here for," he said harshly. "I brought you here to tell you to make me well again. I can't stand this any longer."

"Who gave you the silver preparation? Why don't you see him?" I asked.

"Dr. Lee Wilson gave it to me, and I gave him something. I gave him his chance and he didn't take it, and now I am going to give you yours."

"I am a student," I said. "I know nothing about this condition except in a general way."

"That's the way they all talked when I ran out of money. All of you have a responsibility for what I have suffered and you needn't think you are going to dodge yours. You can cure me if you try hard enough," he said, and then, crazed with fury, he shouted, "Are you going to help me or not?"

The muscles in his arm twitched and jerked as he tightened his hold on his nightstick, lifted it, and glared at me as though he would strike. "I tell you I can't stand it any longer, and I am not going to! I'll . . . I'll . . . ."

It seemed someone other than myself answered. "I will do everything that it is possible to do," I told him. "I'll study every line that has been written on the subject and will do my best to help you."

As he listened, his coat collar sagged somewhat and I got my first real look into his face. All dark and hidden in shadow, it was as harsh as if some wild sculptor had struck his features from a basalt crag. His dark, narrow eyes were burning with hatred. His nose was long, hooked, and sharp; his stubble-covered jaw, clamped. For a mouth there was only a firm slit. My eyes dropped to his enormous hands. Those fingers moved with tendons of steel.

He seemed puzzled. "Why didn't you say so at first if you wanted to help?" he finally said. "I don't know whether to believe you or not. If you will work at it, you can find a way. It ought not to take long."

He seemed to be talking to himself and then he spoke to me.

"Go . . . go look it up. Then you come back to me. Do you hear?" he screamed. "You know where I am. If you don't come . . ." He hesitated. There was something in his voice that made my blood run cold as he continued, "I'll promise you here and now that if you don't come to me, I will come to you. No matter where you are, I will search the earth to find you."

After a moment, without another word, he motioned me back along the path and followed me to the gate. He unlocked it and turned away into the darkness.

I got into my car and started it. Fearing to take time to turn, I drove straight on. When I was a safe distance away, I took out my handkerchief and wiped the cold perspiration from my brow and hands.

Darkness

As I was not returning by the same route I had used in coming, I was soon lost and it took some time to find another road leading back to the city. For nothing in this world would I have passed that yard again!

I was as good as my word. I searched the libraries for literature on the man's condition but found nothing helpful. I asked every professor, every outstanding practitioner whom I met, but they only shook their heads. I talked to chemists and at last satisfied myself that the condition was indeed hopeless. I looked for the name of Dr. Lee Wilson, first in the telephone book and then in the city directory. No such name was listed. I asked the older doctors about him. Yes, they said, they remembered Dr. Wilson. He was dead.

"What caused his death? Was there anything strange about it?" I asked. They did not know.

Time dragged by. When would the man become impatient? What would he do when he realized that I would not return? I had decided going back could do no good. I dared not face him with my failure. I wrote a letter telling him the result of my search and addressed it to the road where he lived, but in a few days it was returned to me marked "Unknown." I expected that the man might call me over the telephone but he did not. I could not erase from my memory his look and the tone of his voice when he said that if I didn't come to him, he would come to me. I made no more night calls and but few in the daytime and those with great caution. I stayed at the hospital most of the time and bolted my door when in my room.

A few more weeks went by and my course was over. It was time for me to leave the city. Shortly before I left, I telephoned to one junkyard after another until I found the one that I had visited.

"No," the office man said, "Barrett is not here now. No, I don't know where he went. It was some time ago. No, he didn't say. One morning when we came in, he just wasn't here. We still owe him some money. If you see him, tell him to come for it."

I thought of the river, but no—not until he had settled with me. I made a guarded check at his home. A new family was occupying the house. No one knew his whereabouts. When I left the city, I requested that the school not give my home address to anyone without first obtaining permission from me.

Even after I had been through the war and had started my own practice, I could not entirely put from my mind the memory of that fearful night. It was the first thing I thought of when the telephone rang after dark. Through those first years, I never walked alone in the shadows. Never did I make a visit without satisfying myself that it could not be he who was behind the call. Gradually I relaxed these precautions, but a vague uneasiness lingered on.

When I saw him, he was much older than I and many years have passed since then—so many that I now know for certain that I need not fear for him any longer. Yet knowing is one thing and feeling is quite another. Deep in my mind he still lives in his prime. For even now as I walk along the streets at night and think that I see a heaviness in the shadow behind a telephone pole, my heart quickens somewhat and my mind pictures the lurking figure of a tall, powerfully built man with his hat brim pulled down, his coat collar held up over his slate-colored face, and his enormous hand gripping a long nightstick as he flattens himself against the pole and bides his time.

The Trip Home

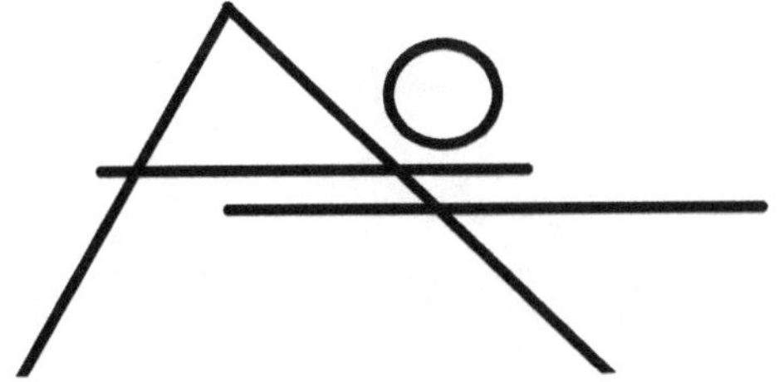

The Trip Home

A nurse opened the door. Standing at the window was a frail woman, looking out across the snow. A strange stillness hung about her. She stood unaware of our presence and apparently unaware of the bleak scene before her yet rapt by it—as if compelled to look forever. I felt the surgeon's hand upon my shoulder, urging me forward, and heard his voice introducing me as a fellow in his clinic accompanying him on his rounds.

She turned. In her blue eyes lay a calmness so unearthly and profound that a moment passed before I became aware that she was holding out her hand to me. For all the white streaks in her hair, her smile was as gentle as that of a child. Her voice was so friendly and so completely lacking in self-consciousness that I was instantly drawn to her and began to have an apprehension for the wan look, which even now several days after her operation, she still bore.

After the nurse prepared the patient, the surgeon examined the site of the operation. As he did so I saw at a glance that she was doomed.

"Well, the incision is all healed and you leave us today, don't you?" he said.

A smile passed over the responsive face. "Everyone has been so kind," she said. "I knew you would cure me if I came in time and you have."

She looked up to him in trusting faith.

I was sorely troubled. I looked to the surgeon for the saving word. There was none. He was a man of handsome and distinguished appearance. Every line, every movement of his body, every glance from beneath those heavy eyebrows carried the suggestion of strength and sureness that had made his name and clinic known to every doctor in the world. His clear gray eyes were studying her face as if to speak. Then his manner changed. With a smile and a slight shake of the head he dismissed her thanks. He spoke of his pleasure in having had her as a patient and told her good-bye.

I followed the surgeon as he moved toward the door. The operation had been palliative. Why had he not told her? Suddenly, as if in answer to my unspoken questions, he stopped and turned to her again.

"Will you do me a favor?" he asked.

"Why, of course," she answered, puzzled. "What can it be?"

"I must go on," he replied, "but I want my young friend to stay and hear the story you told to me the day you came."

She hesitated a moment and then began.

"Well, the first thing I noticed . . ."

"No, it is about yourself that I want him to hear—all of it— just as you told it to me. Tell him where you lived."

"In Alaska," she said, "beyond the river, north of Fairbanks."

"And when you went there," he prompted.

"In 1898."

"And why."

She smiled and then began her story.

"John and I were sweethearts at the university in Seattle. We had planned to work, to save, and to build a white cottage on the Sound. Then one day gold was struck in the Klondike. The papers were filled with stories of fortunes washed out of the streams. It was a chance to avoid long years of labor—a chance to save our youth. We too would go. We bought tickets for the next steamer and were married. All our friends came down to the dock and laughed and waved to us. It was to be our honeymoon. Only a few months and we would be back with the gold!

"It wasn't until we entered the Inside Passage that I realized what it meant—how vast and impersonal was that wilderness and how small and inconsequential was the life of man!" Her smile was gone. She was living those days over again. "I would have turned back but could not. Every moment I bore on—into its vastness.

"The ship would sail through a channel so narrow that I could throw a stone to where the hemlocks dipped their dark branches into the water. Sometimes it was hard to hold our own in the rush of the tide and we were almost dashed against the rocks. Sometimes we would pass an immense glacier. Sometimes a cliff towered so high above the mast that the ship seemed but a toy beside it and our deck was drenched by the spray of the cataract that poured down its face. Then all at once the strait would open out in promise, but it would only lead into some windswept bay. I was little more than a child and it terrified me. The low-lying mist and fog, the great expanse of snow and ice, the spirit of the eternal about it awakened all my primitive fear. Nature seemed so unmindful of our existence.

"Skagway was a city of tents when we arrived. It sheltered us one night and then we pressed on to the gorge. It was there I first saw privation and exhaustion and horror. Seven thousand men toiled through White Pass to the Yukon and down to Dawson that winter."

She paused. "Well, we didn't strike any gold," she continued after a while. "Our stake was gone, and we knew what hunger meant before we gave up the search. We could have come out of another country but not that one. Distances were too great and it was too barren to support life along the way. My husband found work in a mine farther north. We built a cabin. Then our children came and tied us there, but I never called it home. I could never give up the plans we had made or throw off the loneliness that land casts over everyone who sees its vastness and breathes its clear, cold air. I would stand in the door and look across the plains toward my old home three thousand miles away.

"And then those endless nights would come—the stars and the snow and the silence. I feared that I might become an insensible part of it all—of the hush and the solitude and that dreary waste.

"Every grain of gold dust that we could put aside was saved for our return, but there were backsets aplenty and long periods of idleness—times when no work could be done. To step through the door was to be swallowed up, tracks and all, in a blinding storm that cut the face like a lash and turned the world into a wilderness where every moving thing died and became white with the drifting snow."

She waited so long to continue that it was almost as if she had finished. "It was a living death," she said at last in a low tone, "and I wanted life. I wanted life where roses bloom, where birds sang in the spring, where my friends waved to me and loved me, and were glad that I lived.

"Years went by—twenty of them. Then this trouble came and I realized that I must make haste or lie under those stars forever.

"That was a year ago. Once I had a friend with the same trouble. When she finally went to the doctor, he said that it had scattered. He wouldn't operate on her. That was the fear that haunted me.

"My lump slowly grew. I packed and got things ready, but it was a full year before we could sell our cabin and get all the money we needed. Though a blizzard was brewing, we started. It was seventy-two hours by dogsled to Fairbanks. Two days more and we were aboard the steamer in Resurrection Bay.

"At the sight of the bay I was seized again by the great fear I had been fighting off—that it was already too late—that the doctors would put me off on one pretext or another. I suppose it was the still black water and the white slopes rising so precipitously from its edge, and that weird, unearthly light beyond the mountains. It seemed the very dwelling place of death. The rocks to the outlet were black as ink. We were through them and the salt spray was in my face before my courage came again.

"On our trip across the North Pacific we never lost sight of the mountains. The roll of the ship, the tossing of the blue waves thrilled me with the joy of being alive. We sat on the deck for hours, dreaming, watching the long sunsets and the play of colors on the snowy ranges to the east. Everything was flooded with rosy light. It was glorious!

"We shall start life over again in Seattle. We will build in the spruce overlooking the sound. My husband will work in the city and the children can go to school. My life has been like an Arctic night and now the day is coming. I have planned and planned, and oh, I am so happy! I am going home."

The Duffle Bag

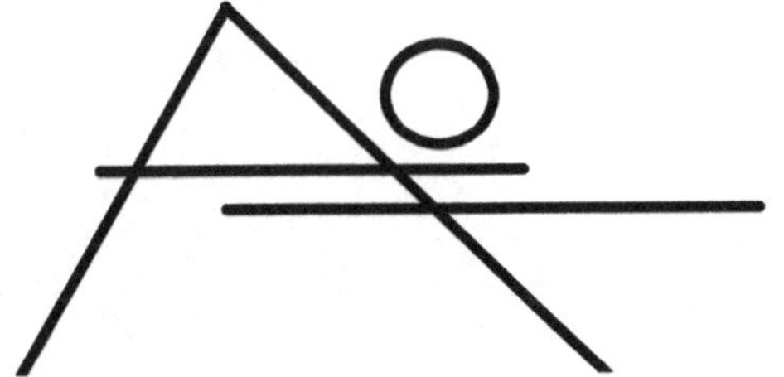

The Duffel Bag

The hospital ship had completed its mission of bringing wounded soldiers from France and had followed the fleet south. We had come through the locks the evening before and for the night laid anchor in Gatun Lake of the Panama Canal.

The sound of rushing feet and a violent knocking on my stateroom door aroused me from a deep sleep.

"Quick, Doctor!" cried the messenger. "A man has gone down at the dock. The divers are bringing him up now. A boat for you is at the gangway."

I sprang from my bunk, pulled my trousers over my pajamas and catching up my socks, shoes, and blouse, raced for the boat. As I jumped in, the boat's bell sounded, and we rapidly moved away from the ship. Hastily I finished my dressing and took my seat in the stern.

I was told that upon arrival at the lake the evening before, the ship's boats had taken a large liberty party ashore. Those who had leave until quarters the next morning had spent the night ashore. In the early morning they had come to the dock to take the first boat back to the ship. A member of this liberty party had fallen into the water.

Though the sun was not yet up, the whole sky was filled with that calm, first light of its approach. The dawn seemed as fresh as the dawn of the earth—a morning for glorious life and not one on which to die. The clear water lay motionless save for the high waves thrown up by our bow that trailed off into the long, diverging ripples of the wake. Here and there thin filmy wisps of vapor still lay upon the surface of the water. Farther back in the bay, small milk-white banks of mist hung motionless. A fish jumped far out in the lake. The verdure along the shore was jewel-like in its overlapping shades, green as only the growth in the tropics can be, and by its reflections made not only twice as great but twice as intense in its coloring.

As we approached the dock, we were hailed by an officer in another boat and instructed to heave to and stand off least our nearer approach interfere with the search.

This boat now came alongside. Its officer was directing the search. He said that as the liberty party, in high spirits, had pushed and shoved and crowded into the boat, a man stepping on its gunwale had lost his footing. He had fallen into the water between the dock and the side of the boat.

"We think that he must have struck his head as he fell," the officer said. "If he came up at all, he came up under the boat or under the dock."

Shortly after the man had gone down, several expert swimmers had stripped and entered the water. Here and there one would come up for a mouthful of air and then swim rapidly downward to explore the bottom of the lake. They were searching not only in the dark shadow under the dock but also some distance out. Other sailors were lying prone on the dock, their heads over its edge, and still others were bending over the gunwales of their boats—all peering into the water. I also bent down and, shading my eyes with my hand, attempted to search the bottom.

The Duffle Bag

In full light and undisturbed, the water was so transparent that the bottom, twenty feet down, seemed much closer. Now, however, in half-light and with refractions due to undulations caused by the movements of the divers, objects lying on the bottom were difficult to identify. I gave up my search.

"The beams of our searchlights were not enough to help much beneath the dock," said the officer. "Now that the sun is coming up, the divers will soon find him."

"Do you know who he is?" I asked.

"The officer of the deck has checked the names of those who have come aboard against the list of those on leave," he replied. "He says the missing man is George Petloff, fireman, third class."

The swimmers were now frantically pushing the search. It is hopeless, I thought. Even if they find him now, it is too late.

Up and down they came and went. Presently there was a large rippling and disturbance, and the head and powerful shoulders of a swimmer broke the water. He was dragging the deathly white form of a man encased in a water-soaked white uniform with its blue scarf.

The coxswain of our boat was ready. One quick tug of his rope spun the flywheel of the motor and we moved up. Now two or three sailors from below and as many from above pushed and pulled the dripping form into the boat.

Quickly the man was turned upon his face and picked up at the hips. Water drained from him onto the bottom of the boat. Several jolts of my fist on the back of his chest dislodged more water from his lungs and there was a gush from his mouth. In a moment the air passages were cleared and dried. Artificial respiration began and the boat raced for the ship.

Upon a pallet laid on the deck of the first-aid room, I continued my efforts. Now another medical officer came to help.

There was no heartbeat. There was no response. We pressed pulse-like over his heart in an attempt to start it— applied oxygen and then took turns with artificial respiration. I would work at it until my arms, shoulders, and back ached. Then the other doctor or a man from the hospital corps would take over the effort.

I was young then and inexperienced. I had heard of success after an unbelievably long time. I didn't know then that after a person hasn't breathed for a minute every second counts—and that after ten minutes resuscitation is practically impossible.

At one time it seemed to me as if George might be getting pinker—that color might be coming into his face. Then again, as I leaned on the operating table while resting and watched while others worked, I finally decided that this was not the case. If there was any pinkness at all, it did not increase but rather faded away.

The engineer officer, who had charge of the firemen, came. It was indeed George, he said. Several of the sailors and firemen who had worked with George came. No one seemed to be very close to him. All they could tell was that he had requested duty on the West Coast and had come aboard the day we left the States.

A drowning man recalls in an instant all the happenings of his life so it is said. An onlooker's mind in such an emergency is also keyed to a high pitch. As I stood and looked down at the form upon the pallet, many and varied pictures of what his life might have been passed through my mind. Each one was rejected.

As for his appearance, his stripped body lay for all to see. He seemed much older than the twenty-four years I had been told was his age. He appeared to be somewhat above average height, though I knew that a person lying down looks longer than he really is. His pallid, bloodless body was so thin that every tug and expansion of the chest by the movements of artificial respiration brought the outline of each of his thin ribs into view. His coarse, brown hair was short from a crew haircut, his face somewhat freckled, his features thin and small—scant would be a good general term with which to describe them. The pupils of his half-closed brown eyes were widely dilated.

Handsome or not, he is everything to someone, I thought, and I pictured a scene of sorrow in some distant home when our message should arrive.

Hopeless it seemed, but I was driven onward by those thoughts.

His body became warm from the electric heater directed toward it—too warm it would seem if judged by the touch of my hand. I knew, however, that this was only surface heat. There was no circulating blood to carry the heat inward.

The cyanosis about his mouth gradually became more marked and dark splotches settled upon his smooth face. I was forced to admit what I had really known all the time—that there was no hope—that George was dead.

I sought the executive officer and together we went to the ship's captain to tell him of our failure. He received our report quietly and sadly.

"You will send the message to the Department," he said to the executive officer. "Tell them that the body was recovered and is in good condition, that after we receive their instructions, we can send it by the first ship going north."

"The Department will notify the next of kin and tell them that without cost to them the body will be shipped and interred anywhere they request," he explained in answer to my question as to who was to tell his people.

"We want him to look as well as possible when they see him," the captain continued. "Please, Doctor, see to it that he is embalmed properly and has on a good uniform."

The day had almost passed when an orderly brought a copy of a radiogram. "Please read and initial, Sir," he said.

"DO NOT SEND BODY STOP BURY THERE STOP," it began.

I could scarcely read the rest of the message, which dealt at length with instructions for sending George's money and possessions. I was stunned by its callous, grasping words.

His people care nothing for him, it is his property that they want, I thought.

"This sheet also, Sir," said the messenger, handing me a directive from the executive officer.

"Immediately after burial," it read, "in company with the two officers named herein, you shall make a complete list of all property formerly owned by George Petloff, fireman, third class. Sign the list in the presence of one another and send the same to the executive officer. You shall further see that these belongings are properly packed and labeled by the master-at-arms and sent ashore for shipment no later than two hours before sailing time."

"When do we sail?" I asked.

"At nine o'clock tomorrow morning, Sir," answered the orderly.

"Please find out when he is to be buried and let me know. I want to be there," I said to him.

"The burial party is preparing to go ashore now, Sir," he replied.

A little later I stood with a handful of men at George's open grave. A sudden storm had come. The few words spoken by the chaplain were torn into shreds and blown away as they came from his lips. They were inaudible to me. Dark, ominous clouds and a few drops of rain told of the deluge that was to come. The service was rapidly concluded. The riflemen fired their blank cartridges into the air and all returned to the ship—all but George.

As we came aboard, the darkness of the storm and of approaching night was becoming blended with that of my own spirit. The bright lights could not help.

My mind now turned to the executive officer's orders—the tabulation of George's possessions. His relatives had inquired about them with so much interest.

What can they be? I wondered.

The story of a life is often told by the things a man has treasured—the fortune that he has amassed, a work of art, or a locket with its photograph or wisp of hair.

I called my committee together and asked that George's effects be sent to the first-aid room.

The master-at-arms brought in a duffel bag. I stood, pencil and paper pad in hand, as the contents of the bag were poured out upon the tile deck where its former owner's body had lain a few hours before.

I made the list of George's possessions as the master-at-arms drew them aside, one by one, and an officer turned over some of the articles with his foot.

First, I listed the few well-worn and somewhat dingy clothes and then, item by item, the following:

1 safety razor

2 razor blades

1/3 tube shaving cream

1 toothbrush

1 comb

43¢ in cash

1 knife with one broken and one good blade

1/2 pack cigarettes (have been wet)

3 souvenir shells with names and scenes of seaports stamped in color upon them

and that was all.

The Temple

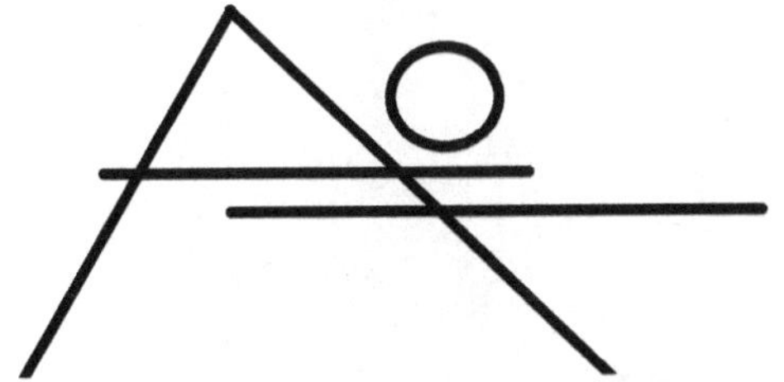

The Temple

There is but one temple and that is the body of man.

Novalis

I strolled about the lush, shady grounds, gazed at the distant views, and walked upon the white-columned portico and on into the stately hall of the building which I was considering for conversion into a private hospital. The building and all of its surroundings would be a most pleasant place in which to spend my life—a perfect setting for a hospital. I resolved then and there to carry the enterprise through. At the same time, while I was under the spell of the beauty about me, came the idea of dedicating my life to the task. Here I would do the finest, the most conscientious, work of which I was capable. Here my dealings with humanity would be in selflessness and purity of heart.

The building has the lofty attributes of a temple, I thought. In that moment a quotation from Novalis came to my mind, and I realized that the temple is a human body, that a building can never be one. Glancing upward in the hall, I saw a panel where the quotation should go.

A little later a friend made a plaque of brass, lettered the words upon this, and placed it in the panel. There it remained for the life of the institution—more than a quarter of a century.

The quotation set the tone for the hospital. For me it stood as a reminder of that first moment of high purpose and idealism. For all it was an ever-present source of comfort and inspiration. It gave, in our minds, a dignity and transcendent value to the humblest human being who came for aid. It made of our profession a higher calling than it would have been. It made of the hospital a hallowed ground. It made us feel that we were not alone while watching and serving through the long night, going into a patient's room and then coming out again, walking in the halls, waiting—waiting for nature to reassert itself. The quotation ever reminded us of the Spirit that dwells in that temple, of that force of nature which the Divine Hand created—the force that produces the body, nurtures it, strives to repair its injuries and to preserve its life. It kept this marvelous force in view. It caused me to stand before it in awe and contemplative wonder as over the years, in almost every type of injury and disease, in thousands of cases, I thought of and pondered its power. Many times, I mentioned this miraculous force to some patient—at times in some detail.

Lee McConnell, a strong young man, had come into the hospital on a rather unusual mission. He had come to thank me again for my services and to show me his right hand, now well, which a year before had been rendered useless by a severe injury of the wrist.

The day of the injury had been a stormy one. The light rain that had begun in the afternoon and slightly melted snow had turned to sleet as a cold wind moved in at sundown. The temperature continued to fall and soon all that lay without was covered with a glistening sheet of ice.

Mr. McConnell, his wife, and two small children had that morning driven into an adjoining county to visit Mrs. McConnell's parents and were on their way home when the sleet storm struck. No chains could hold upon the ice. Mr. McConnell tore up his lap robe and wove it into the chains. His car limped home.

The babies were tired and hungry. The milk, which had been delivered earlier in the day, was still in the box at the gate. Mr. McConnell cautiously descended the kitchen steps and made his way to the box. The milk was frozen, but it could be thawed. With a bottle in each hand, he slowly returned up the path. As he stepped upon the glassy surface of the steps, his feet shot from under him. The bottle in his right hand struck the concrete tread and his right wrist came violently down upon the jagged edge of the broken bottle. He knew enough to seize the injured wrist with his left hand, to thrust his left thumb into the terrible wound, and to press firmly upon the spouting artery. This stopped the chief loss of blood and saved his life. He was able to maintain this hold until a nearby doctor, summoned over the telephone, could arrive. The doctor applied a tourniquet above the elbow, where the single bone allows the main artery to be compressed.

The trek over ten miles of icy roads to the hospital began. It was the middle of the night when he was finally laid on the operating table.

I examined the wound and found that every flexor tendon in the right wrist had been severed—two to each of the fingers and two to the thumb—as well as others to the fascia and to the wrist bones. The radial artery had been cut. The medial nerve had been divided. This nerve injury had resulted in a numbness in the fingers it normally supplied. The hand was helpless; not a finger could be closed.

It was three hours by the clock from the time the operation was started until the last stitch was taken, the dressing applied, and the patient returned to his room.

The wound quickly healed. The hand became stronger and yet stronger and the patient was discharged from my care.

Now, after one year to the day, Mr. McConnell in his delight and gratitude had returned to show me the hand and to express his thanks. To all appearances the hand was normal. The transverse scar on the wrist coincided with and resembled the bracelet folds so closely as to be almost indistinguishable from them. Mr. McConnell opened and closed his fingers. They had their full and normal movement.

"They are as strong as they have ever been," he said. The numbness had disappeared and, in every respect, the sensation in his hand and fingers was normal.

He spoke of his gratitude to me, of what a fine surgeon he considered me to be.

"When I came to you, I thought I was ruined," he said. "I didn't think anyone on earth could repair the injury so that I could use the hand again. It is wonderful—a miracle!"

"Yes," I replied. "It is a miracle. The miracle, however, lies in what nature did after I failed so miserably to complete the repair. Sit down and let me tell you about it."

I sat at my desk. He took a chair across from me.

"When you first came, the hand looked rather hopeless," I began. "First, I tied the larger vessels. I then cleansed the wound as best I could and swabbed it with a mild antiseptic, one that would kill many germs but by no means all of them. Next, the proximal end of a tendon was picked up and the distal end of the same tendon searched for, found, and sutured to it. The torn covering was then drawn over the tendon and loosely caught together here and there with fine catgut sutures. This repair was continued until all tendons were repaired.

"Next, I repaired the nerve. The two ends of its severed trunk were found. In general structure a nerve trunk may be likened to a telephone cable. Its heavy, fibrous sheath wraps, protects, and supports its bundle of filaments. These filaments are projections from the nerve cells located near the spinal cord and, like tiny, insulated wires, run from these cells to their end organs in the muscles and sensory buds. In the cross section of the nerve trunk that I was holding, I could see that there were more filaments in some parts of the field than there were in others. I matched the two irregular patterns and caught the fibrous tissue together with fine sutures.

"A few sutures drew the connective tissue beneath the skin together; and then with silk, I sutured the skin.

"There stood my repair—crude, full of knots."

"Don't be so modest, Doctor," Mr. McConnell broke in. "It was good enough for me."

"No, it wasn't," I told him. "I am not quite through. Let me finish what I started to say.

"My repair had been made solely for the purpose of holding the structure together until the body could do its work. At the longest, the deep sutures could last only two or three weeks. The union was so weak that a strong handshake would have pulled them out and destroyed my work. The repair had been made, I believe, as well as was humanly possible; yet, in comparison with the repair that was to follow, it was a makeshift—a sorry job.

"Upon the forearm and hand, I molded some plaster splints, put it all in a sling, went to bed and to sleep, and passed the real repair of the injury on to that force capable of making it.

"There in the dark, under the cast—yes, in the middle of the arm—the body cells, each with a mind of its own, realized what had happened. Like an army of ants, they went to work. Each cell knew what was expected of it and each performed its task.

"Though all the various phenomena of repair moved along together, I shall have to speak of one system; and then another as I give you an outline of what took place."

Mr. McConnell was interested now. His attention hung on every word I spoke.

"When your radial artery was cut," I continued, "and the tissues beyond were deprived of most of their blood supply, a rather remarkable thing happened. All the smaller vessels connecting these tissues with neighboring arteries enlarged to bring in the needed blood. That didn't just happen. It was nature's way of bringing additional blood to these tissues. In the cut vessels of the injured area, the complicated process of the clotting of blood took place. Other vessels dilated temporarily to speed circulation and repair. Their walls became more permeable and through them seeped serum, which, clotting into fibrin, entangled germs and immobilized the structures. Through all this time the bacteria were fighting for their very lives. They were trying to break through this entanglement, to multiply, to spread. They were doing their best to melt these clots and to kill you with their poisons. Your body, in answer, inaugurated a strange and, as far as details are concerned, unknown reaction—that of the production of antitoxins and antibodies to neutralize the poisons. In the bone marrow chiefly, an increased number of white blood cells were produced. These entered the blood stream and were borne to the troubled area. Pushing into the tissues, they seized and devoured the bacteria. They carried away the dead cells and detritis and secreted lycins to dissolve my sutures.

"Cells at all of the cut surfaces, stimulated in some unknown way, were now undergoing the complicated process of division. One cell, dividing, made two. Each of these in turn made two more; so that soon the gaps across the tendons, their sheaths, the nerve trunk, the skin, and all the other structures were filled with young, interlacing cells.

"Clots in the vessels were first fixed and then replaced by invading cells. Mosaic-like cells that lined the blood vessels divided and covered these organized clots. Strong fibers were woven into the tendons. Rough and protruding bumps and edges were everywhere removed. Over the raw surface of the tendons grew cells that formed a smooth, glistening covering and secreted an oily fluid so that the tendons might glide smoothly. When a sufficient number of cells had been produced, another unknown factor took command and the cells stopped dividing.

"This control—this ability of the body to check the division of cells—is, so far as man is concerned, the most important fact in nature. Without it there would be no organized life. How many millions of dollars have been poured out and how many years of labor of thousands of the best minds of the world have been spent in the effort to understand this one phenomenon, and still its explanation is not in sight!

"Oh yes," I said to my patient, "I almost forgot one thing but the body didn't. Your hand would soon be normal save for the numbness in some fingers and the slightly impaired motion of the tip of the thumb and index finger. To a casual examiner, the united nerve trunk would, at that time, have appeared normal but it was not. The distal ends of the filaments which carried the nerve impulses, having been cut off from their source of nourishment, had died and been absorbed, leaving minute canals running through the tubes of insulating material. The nerve cells at the spinal cord began to push down the cut ends of the filaments. Each of these, feeling about, found its own opening and began to grow down its own canal. Slowly the nerve filaments advanced. As months passed, the sensory filaments reached the skin of the fingers and the motor filaments came to their muscles. Each filament now reactivated its own end organ, and sensation and movement returned.

"It would require many volumes to record what scientists have observed in nature's repair of the body, but still they know little of what really takes place. As each phenomenon is explained, each veil drawn aside, another, like the veil of Isis[1], covers what is beyond."

Lee McConnell's eyes had turned from me. He was following thoughts of his own—lost in abstraction.

"All we have ever seen," I continued, "has been but a glimpse of the material forms, of the cells as they have

---

1. William Winwood Reade, *The Veil of Isis or Mysteries of the Druids*, (Newcastle Publishing company, 1992),126. The veil of Isis which "concealed all the mysteries and learning of the past."

performed their functions; has been but a glance toward that mysterious realm of life, intangible and shadowy, that lies within.”

“Yes,” I said, “this repair was marvelous—a miracle.”

He sat for a while, then arose and, still in deep thought, walked quietly out.

He had not said good-bye, nor had he looked my way. In the presence of the real doctor, I had been forgotten.

The Stain

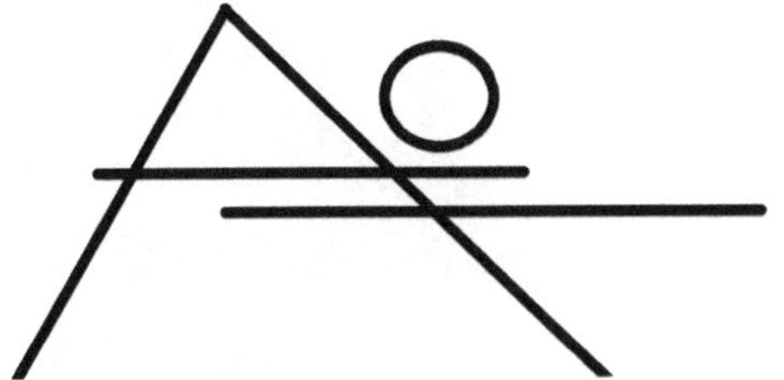

The Stain

The rough, overgrown path, still wet with dew, led to the old house where Mildred Kemp, my young secretary, lived with her elder sister. The dilapidated house came into view. The sister was standing on the porch, her face white and drawn. She did not speak nor did she move to go in with me. Instead, as one in a dream, she pointed down the hall to the door of Mildred's room.

The moment I saw Mildred I knew she was not a patient I could treat. The light of reason had fled from her eyes. She took no notice of my entry nor of what I tried to say to her. Rapidly, never pausing for an instant, she paced back and forth. She talked incessantly, incoherently. I left her and returned to the porch. There her sister gave me an account of the night before. What she said made me all the more certain that Mildred should have expert observation and treatment.

I explained this necessity and, summoning all the tact at my command, advised that she be committed to a nearby mental institution. After receiving the sister's sanction, I telephoned to the asylum and made the necessary arrangements.

A little later I rode in the ambulance with Mildred and the guards and, after her admission to the institution, waited until the preliminary examination had been completed. As I had feared, the prognosis was all but hopeless.

Leaving Mildred and the asylum, I began my walk back across the fields. My mind retraced each related incident of the few months that I had known her.

When Mildred entered my employment, she had just finished her course in a business college. She was what might be called a slip of a girl, somewhat above average in height, very thin, with a slight awkwardness as if she had just finished her rapid growth. She was very fair—her hair a little browner than light gold. In her blue eyes was a certain look of abstraction that I did not understand at the time.

"Please let me try. I need the work," she pled when I expressed a doubt that she had the strength to fill the position. Her childlike appeal made it impossible for me to refuse her.

She was reticent when I made any remark or asked any question of a personal nature. No word of her past, her present, or her future ever fell from her lips.

This very aloofness may have played a part in her undoing, I now thought, for it had discouraged the conversations and closer associations which might have given an insight as to what was taking place.

Though she never smiled, Mildred was always pleasant and agreeable. She displayed a certain air of detachment as she went about her work—answering the telephone, greeting patients, making appointments, collecting accounts, writing letters.

She took these tasks almost too seriously. She was a little too meticulous. There was an almost tremulous fear of failure, as I remembered now. She was anxious to please, to confer a favor, but she would never accept one in return.

"Oh no, Sir! I like to help you," she would say to my apology for keeping her overtime in an emergency.

But, when we had finished and I said that I should like to take her home, she would thank me and put me off with one excuse or another.

The busiest days, with their multitude of details requiring nerve force and stamina, were the very days I had the least opportunity to notice her work or to observe how she endured the strain. The first suggestion of trouble was the tone of her sister's voice when Mildred failed to report for work that morning.

"Oh, why did I employ her when I doubted her strength, even for a moment? Why did I allow myself to be persuaded? Why did I not see that she was breaking?" These were the questions that kept coming to my mind.

Filled with self-reproach, I reached the unpainted shell of a house with its thin, worn floors and walls of crumbling plaster. It made me think of the haunted houses of my childhood, yet Mildred had called it home.

The sister still stood upon the porch just as I had left her. I repeated what the doctors had told me and then said that I wondered if the fault could be mine.

"No, Doctor," she said in a dead and hopeless voice. "You were lovely to her. It goes farther back than that."

I looked inquiringly at her.

After a few moments she began to speak again: "This kind of thing is not new to us. We have always lived on this farm near the state asylum—and for a reason. My father was a victim of cyclic insanity. My earliest remembrances are of times of sadness—of those times when he was confined in the institution.

"When normal, he was a devoted parent working hard to provide a living for his family. However, when the wheel had turned full circle and, as the doctors said, the red flag came to the surface, he was utterly irresponsible.

"Usually, he could tell when the trouble was coming on and would give himself up to be restrained until he was normal again. At other times he had no warning and we cowered before a dangerous madman until the officers arrived to take him away".

"All through our childhood," she continued, "our father lived first with us and then behind those gray walls.

"One winter, when Mildred was about nine, a time of comparative happiness was ending in apprehension and strain. We were fearful of trouble and it came. Cries of alarm and a commotion in the hall awoke us in the middle of the night. Then all was quiet and we heard my mother's pleading voice. We all ran downstairs. My father had brought in a shotgun that he had secretly obtained and kept hidden in the barn.

My mother was holding on to it—trying to keep him from using it. 'Don't come here. Run!' she cried to us.

"Of the terror-stricken children, Mildred alone knew what to do. Barefooted, clad only in her nightgown, she ran for help—out into the winter night and across the fields. The rest of us stayed huddled in the living room. We could hear our mother's panting as she struggled with my father. Sometimes he was quiet and she pleaded with him to turn the gun loose. Then again he struggled for it.

"An age passed before there came the sounds of shouting and of rushing feet, and guards from the asylum burst in. 'I won't go back,' my father screamed. He jerked the gun from mother and with it in hand raced up the stairs into a room and locked the door.

"The guards tried the door, attempted to reason with him, begged him to put the gun aside and give himself up to safety. Failing this, they brought a ladder. While some attempted to attract his attention at the door, others began to force the window.

"We could hear him move above us—hear him cock the gun. Then came the deafening report and my father's falling body shook the house."

She stood, inanimate now save for the slight movement of her hands as she caught together and twisted the tips of her cold, blanched fingers.

She started to speak again, hesitated, and finally said: "Yes, I will . . . I will show it to you."

"What?" I asked hoarsely.

For an answer she led the way in and opened the door to the living room. I started to enter, glanced up, and stopped—struck motionless with horror—my eyes fixed upon a great stain in the ceiling—a dark, savage, unmistakable red—which through the years had lent its awful coloring to everything beneath.

The Burden

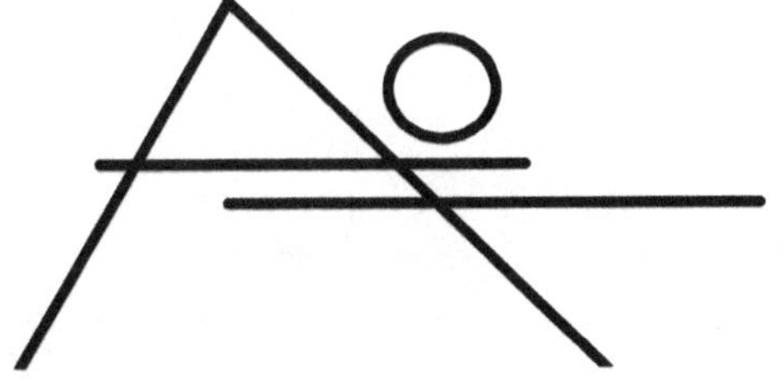

The Burden

The practice of medicine requires a high degree of self-consecration. He who would put self-interest, convenience, pleasure, his friends, or even his own family before his duty to his patients is unworthy of the name of doctor. Yet, this doctor is still a human being, with all the weaknesses, desires and emotions of one. The personal sacrifices that he must make over the years—the giving up for the higher aim all the little joys and things that he loves—gradually draw him from the usual paths of life, isolate him, set him apart from his fellow man, give him many heartaches, leave him with many longings, and make of his profession at times a cross—and one not easy to bear.

I first became aware of the kind of life that I was to live when, as a young man, I was doing surgery in a hospital connected with a large navy yard.

It was winter and night was falling. The yard whistle blew as I walked from the administration building towards the wards where lay several very sick patients. All at once I became conscious of the difference between the life of a doctor and that of the thousands of workmen who, having put aside their tools, now streamed from the shops—free until the morrow—free to go home to their families and their other interests. I glanced at the sinking sun. Far into that night I would be on the wards, anxiety and care my only companions.

The day came when I left military service and started into private practice. At first, I had few patients and therefore more leisure time in which to cultivate and enjoy a number of friendships which I now formed and which meant a great deal to me. As I was of a very responsive, affectionate nature, one who loved his friends and was loyal to them, never requiring anything from them but their affection; the friendships I made were deep and lasting ones. It was through this rather brief period that I had some of the happiest, most memorable experiences of my life.

Soon the demands of a growing practice began to bring this phase of life to a close. Then came the time when after planning to attend some function with my friends or family I would have to forego the anticipated pleasure. I would start to play a game of golf, only to see a caddy coming from the clubhouse, a white slip of paper in his hand, summoning me to leave the foursome and return to the hospital to cope with some emergency. I would accept a dinner invitation and be forced to be late or to telephone at the last minute and say that I could not come. These incidents disturbed me. Gradually I withdrew from almost all social life.

The years of grueling labor began—years that allowed no day—I might almost say no hour—of rest. I saw my friends seldom now, but I loved them still and held them in a different way. I had managed to bring them over into a new relationship, quieter than the old one but comfortable and highly prized. That is, I managed to keep all but one—one of the dearest. His loss came about through an inopportune demand upon me by a patient, causing a delay in carrying out my pledge to my friend.

The tragedy that followed hurt me so much that I never again went into that paradise where I had been happy with him. I put my gun and rod and reel aside for the last time. Even now, after all these years, I cannot think of that day without the keenest pain.

I shall call him Thomas Nash. Our friendship, developing slowly at first, became very close before the two years I knew him had passed. I met him one fall, rather casually it seemed, at the home of a mutual friend. A short time afterwards I was pleased to receive a letter inviting me to bring my gun and spend a night with him at a hunting lodge only few miles from his home—about thirty-five from my own. I eagerly accepted the invitation.

On the afternoon named, having followed directions, I came at length to an inlet in the forest and drove slowly along the narrow, rocky road I was to take many times during the next two years and then no more. The road lay beneath the swamp maples with their riot of color and between and around great clumps of rhododendron. I could hear the sound of a waterfall nearby. All at once the view opened out into a scene of almost breathtaking beauty—a great, wooded basin girt round with mountains. The clubhouse, a lodge made of large poplar logs with the bark still on, stood just ahead. To the side of the lodge flowed a stream, a clear rivulet that rushed and broke into white foam on the rocks and then widened out into a broad pool below.

As I drove up, Thomas Nash came from the lodge to welcome me. I had forgotten exactly how he looked, though I remembered his voice. I now saw again that he was tall, slender, and lithe.

There isn't an ounce of fat on him, I thought. The grace and lightness and ease in his walk belied his age. He must have been near fifty. His composure, his strong sun-tanned face and the level gaze of his light gray eyes all marked the skilled woodsman I knew him to be. His hand was thin and firm. The most unusual things about him, however, were his smile and his voice. His smile, while slight and quiet, had a brightness about it not often seen and his voice carried a timbre that I had never heard elsewhere. It was as musical as a freshly rosined violin bow drawn across the strings.

We stood for a while, looking first at the distant view and then at the great hemlocks that grew about the house and here and there along the stream. He seemed very pleased that I thought it so beautiful.

"The rivulet is called Shining Creek," he said, and as it sparkled in the sun, I could not think of a more appropriate name. Within the clubhouse a great log fire was blazing on the rough stone hearth. I was introduced to the rest of the party. They all called one another by their first names and at once called me by mine. They were a jolly, joking, laughing crowd, but none of them was as attractive as my host.

He seated me before the fire, made several provisions and suggestions for my comfort and, after disappearing, soon returned with some refreshments.

A rather unusual display of courtesy, I thought, amid a group of men like these. I later found that such thoughtful acts were not at all unusual for him.

The Burden

The room was large, the ceiling sloping upward with the rafters of the roof. Around the wall were mounted fish and the heads and antlers of deer. In what was called the Amen Corner a number of pieces of cloth stenciled with names and dates were tacked to the wall. These were the shirttails of members each of whom had had a fair shot and missed his buck. Several bearskins were scattered over the floor. On a board of the floor I saw the outline of a large fish and, when I remarked upon it, one of the men told me that it was the outline of the largest trout ever caught in Shining Creek. A member of the club had caught it a few years before and traced its profile in pencil. By a vote of the club, it had been outlined with a knife.

There were some good cooks in the party and a considerable stock of venison from the kill of the morning, as well as beef and ham brought in for those who did not like game.

That night some good storytellers were among the group gathered around the fire—one especially good one. Happenings of the countryside, little everyday things, told vividly by him, took on a new meaning. Tom did not join in the storytelling, but he led the singing with his wonderful tenor voice.

Most of the party slept in bunks in the big room, before the open fire. Tom and I slept in a little room across the end of the large one.

"If you are like I am," he said to me, "you can't get any rest in a room where everybody is boiling coffee and smoking all night." Tom did not smoke, which may have partly accounted for the whiteness of his fine, strong teeth.

The next morning, while still dark, Tom awoke. He was the first up. After a standing-up and walking-about breakfast of bacon and scrambled eggs and black coffee, during which equipment was got in order and final plans were made, the party filed out. I was to go with Tom to a ridge called Raven Crest. When we left the clubhouse, he handed me a paper-wrapped package of sandwiches and an apple. These were to be my lunch.

As we reached the crest, a regular gale was blowing. The timber was swaying and lashing its branches to and fro.

"It's a bad day for a hunt," said my companion. "No dog can pick up a scent in a wind like this."

We stayed on the ridge until daylight. Not a sound did we hear save the roaring of the storm in the trees.

At Tom's suggestion we returned to camp and shot at tin cans placed on posts. Later we sat by the fire and talked. I was so interested in what he had to say and enjoyed the quiet restfulness of the day so much that I was really glad the hunt had turned out as it had.

One by one the tired hunters straggled in through the long afternoon. None had seen any game.

The party now began to break up. The deer that had been killed the day before were divided and the hunters insisted that I take a quarter. As my host walked with me to my car, I tried to thank him, to tell him what the day had meant to me.

Then he spoke. "Somehow I feel that you look upon all this in a different way from the others," he said. "As much as they enjoy it, they don't love it as I do. I believe that you could. I often come here alone to spend the night. I intend to come back this weekend. Can't you come to be with me? I'd like to show you what we have here."

Of course, I went. When I got there, I found that he had planned a trip and had prepared a blanket roll with provisions for each of us. It was to be a tramp along the ledge at the outer boundary of the basin. We would spend the night at the gap, Tom said.

All that afternoon we walked along the faint path that ran through the virgin balsams upon the mountain ridge. Soft, yellowish-green moss covered the ground and blanketed our footfalls. It lay upon every fallen tree, every fallen limb, and ran up the trunks of those most beautiful of all the evergreens. Occasionally one could see out through the trees and down into the blue sky and the white, floating clouds. At dusk we came to a grassy saddle across the ridge—the gap. A bold, clear spring ran from beneath a large stone.

In the clearing was a sloping shelter of bark, a half roof. Some of the hunters had left it, Tom said. Under his guidance we cut boughs from the balsams and, overlapping them in such a way that the butts were down and the tips up, paved the lean-to and upon this spread our blankets.

"An Indian feather bed," he called it.

A large fire at the open side of our shelter gave us a place to cook our bacon on pointed sticks and make our coffee, as well as affording us light and warmth against the chill of night.

We sat upon our blankets and talked. Tom told me how he had known the basin since childhood, how he had at last come to buy it and had organized a club of twelve of his friends, selling each a share at cost. He hoped that they would keep the tract for their children and for his. He had a son of high school age. That night he talked about the college to which he planned to send him in a couple of years and the career of which he dreamed for him. Tom wanted his share in the club to go to him.

"There is a provision that goes with the sale of the shares," Tom said, "that if anyone wishes to sell his share, he must sell it back to me. In that way I can control the membership during my lifetime, although I have never resold a share to anyone unless the entire club approved." He went on to say that there was now a vacancy and with the permission of the other members he was offering this to me.

I told him of my appreciation, how I would like nothing better, but that I had just started practice and really could not afford the price which he had named—a price very low indeed for a twelfth interest in that magnificent property.

"Do you want it? That is the question and the only one," he said. "If you do, you can pay for it when and how you choose."

It was settled that I would pay one-third down, one-third in one year, and the remainder two years from the date I would receive the deed.

"If you cannot meet the payments, all you will have to do is to say so," he told me. "I know you will pay me when you can."

Throughout that next year I often went to the club. Sometimes I could not go just when I planned, but I managed to get in many trips. I never went without making sure that Tom could go. As for him, every time a special occasion arose, he would write to ask me to come. He and I were often there alone, and we stayed pretty well together whether others were there or not.

Many things of interest and beauty came up. These highlights left a lasting memory with me.

One was the time we cut the bee tree. Tom had found it by watching the flight of the bees as they left the stream. We all got stung, but we filled our pails with wild honey.

Another was the morning when, at sunrise, he took me into the poplar flat in the upper part of the basin. Here great, straight, smooth-barked trunks of the poplars rose from their bed of ferns and, extending skyward to the thick canopy of green leaves far above, they stood like columns in some vast house of worship. The whole air was dripping with dew and filled with fog through which struck long, bright shafts of light from the rising sun. There was everywhere the smell of the moist earth and presently, the distant bell-like note of the wood thrush.

One morning, still in its blackness, the rapturous song of a bird awoke us. It came from the small clearing above the lodge. The whole earth seemed to pulse and vibrate and then overflow with the heavenly swell—higher and higher—yet sustained.

"What is it?" I asked Tom when I heard him raise himself upon his elbow to listen.

"I don't know," he said. "I have heard it only once before myself. Then I thought it might be some bird of passage, but an old woodsman told me that it was the robin—that the robin has two songs." The song continued. Then the first faint light of dawn came. The chirping of the lesser voices started and the beautiful strain ceased.

It was Tom's eye that always spotted the squirrel high among the brown leaves. Often, when he wanted me to shoot first, it would take some time for him to point the squirrel out to me.

Then there was the day he caught the trout. At the club there had been a regular pattern for fishing. The members would start at the lodge and fish upstream for a mile or more, through several fine pools, and finish up at the largest pool of all, below a waterfall. We called it the Blue Pool. A winding road had been cut to this point and there a car would be waiting to bring the fishermen back to camp. I, for one, had very indifferent success with my fishing. There were the usual instructions and advice about not wearing white shirts and straw hats, not letting the fish see you, not allowing your shadow to fall on the pool. I tried them all, but my catch did not improve. I was told the old one about catching a fish and cutting it open to examine and try matching the flies it had been eating. Just how this first fish was to be caught was not very clear.

One beautiful day in the spring, Tom and I were alone at the club. Wearing his old fishing hat with the bright-colored flies in the band, Tom came up to where I sat on the porch.

"Get your rod and flies," he said. "I am going to show you how to catch trout."

We drove to the Blue Pool and began where we had always finished. Tom selected a fly closely resembling one fluttering above the stream. He then showed me how to hold the rod and cast the fly. He repeated the demonstration several times.

"Now!" he said. "The first thing you have to do is to go where the fish are and where they haven't been frightened."

He led the way straight up the difficult, rocky bluff beside the falls, and then, stooping low, almost on tiptoe he slipped along the stream. I followed. Presently we came to several large, moss-covered logs that lay across our way. Tom crouched still lower and crept up to the logs, making signs that I should continue to follow and make no sound. Slowly, cautiously, we raised our heads and peeped over the logs. The pool was thirty feet across, fresh, limpid, and filled with moving lights that reflected the colors playing upon its surface and the cascade at its upper edge. At the foot of the falls a number of large trout were feeding. One trout of the school had a white scar upon its back.

"Do you see the one with the white mark?" Tom whispered. "I will catch that one for you."

Up and back came the rod. Tom cast his fly in the shadow of the pool's edge—a few feet from the school. Several fish turned from the falls, separating and spreading out as they did so. Back came the fly, above and behind us, and, looping in a long sinuous movement without pause or abrupt change of direction, it then swung out over the pool and drifted down to the water. Cautiously, the trout swam toward the lure, which Tom now slowly drew and skipped upon the water.

"If he gets it in his mouth, he will spit it out," Tom whispered.

The fish made a slight and guarded rush. Just before it reached the fly, Tom raised his forearm, and the fly came out of the water. Back again, high in the air, it seemed to float, then, under the low-hanging branches on the far side of the pool it ever so lightly touched the water directly before the marked fish. There came the white flash of spray and the gleaming side of the fish as it struck. With a slight lifting movement, Tom set the hook. A brief struggle ensued, and then he swung the trout before me.

Before using his hooks, Tom always bent the barbs down with a pair of pliers. He now wet his hands and eased the hook from the fish's mouth.

"Do you want him?" he asked. When I shook my head, he said, "I will let some of the others catch him again," and slid the fish into the water below the logs.

Standing there that day, it would seem almost impossible that such a friendship could end as it did. Yet the forces had already been set in motion to bring it to its tragic close.

One was my growing practice. Now I could not leave it with the same freedom I formerly had. I could not attend the annual, all-member hunt that fall. Sometimes I would make a date with my friend which I could not keep.

The second factor was worldwide in its scope. It was the Great Depression of the early thirties. Spreading its mantle of fear over the land, it paralyzed men's actions and stole their reason.

Tom was not the man to trouble his friends with his misfortunes; but as the stock market, built on speculation, broke and came down like a house of cards, all values fell and bank after bank closed, including the one with which he dealt. No one who looked into his face could fail to see the effect all this had upon him. A mutual acquaintance told me that Tom had plunged in the market and had lost a fortune.

I was powerless to help him. Although now I had a rapidly growing practice, my patients had, during those days, very little money with which to pay a doctor's bill. I had, however, met my payments for my share in the club and was saving and looking forward to the final one sometime away.

One day I received a visit from Tom. He was tremulous and nervous. He told me that he had met serious reversals, that he could hope to keep but little of his former wealth, and that the thing that hurt him most was to see his son expecting and preparing to go off to school when there was no money to send him. Tom said that he had set his heart upon his son's entry into the university that coming fall and that he felt he had failed him. He asked me if I could make the payment for my share in the club ahead of time in order that his son might have the funds to matriculate.

I did not have the money to make the payment, nor the collateral through which a loan could be negotiated. I told him, however, that there was some money due me which I would try to collect and if I could get it, I would be glad to give it to him—that I would have to let him know.

My debtor promised to pay me, and I sent this message to Tom. When the time came, however, the money was not forthcoming—probably through no fault of my debtor. I relayed this disappointing news to my friend and asked the latest date that his son could matriculate. I told him that I would redouble my efforts. Later, from another source I received a definite promise of the money and at once wrote Tom that I felt the money was in sight and that he could expect me to come to his house with it by three o'clock on the date he had mentioned.

The day came. I got the money and put it in my pocket. Though I had purposely scheduled no surgery, it seemed that everything happened to delay my departure. There was an unusual number of sick patients to be seen and, in addition, emergency surgery that had to be done. Finally, I came down the hospital steps, already late, only to meet a man with a fractured arm on his way to see me.

I followed him back into the hospital. There were the x-rays to wait for and, as it was a bad fracture, the anesthetist and cast room to alert. I set the arm and fixed it with a molded splint.

Free at last, I began the drive to the home of my friend, thirty miles away.

When I reached the village and drove up to his house, I saw a number of men and women standing in the street, the yard and on the porch. After stopping my car and getting out, I inquired about the reason for the crowd.

Only a half hour before, someone told me, Tom had put the muzzle of his gun in his mouth and pressed the trigger.

"It was like him to make a good job of it once he started," said my informer.

"You can't help, Doctor," said another sadly.

It was all too true. I could but hand to his widow the money, now a vain offering, and utter my still more vain regrets.

I was one of Tom's pallbearers. The procession turned toward the mountains and wound along that now all-too-familiar road. It stopped at the foot of a high knoll overlooking the valley he had loved so well. Always in my mind was the memory of what he had been to me, always the thought that he might be living had I arrived on time.

It was a steep hill, and the casket was heavy, but the real burden as I stumbled along was the weight that lay in my heart.

The Getaway

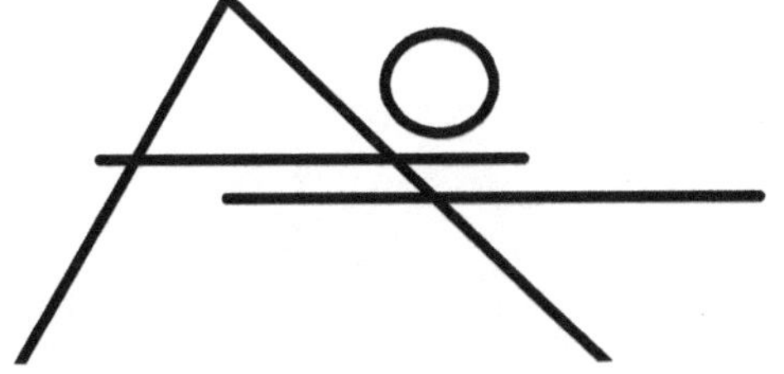

The Getaway

The area around the ambulance entrance of the hospital was filled with cars, some with their headlights burning. The bright beam of a police car's spotlight, cocked at a crazy angle, streamed upward into the night, intensifying, and giving a dramatic air to the blackness.

As I alighted from my car, I saw groups of people standing here and there. I spoke to the policemen as I passed them in the hall. I knew several personally—fine, young men, healthy and strong. They indeed seemed to represent the majesty of the law with their neat blue uniforms, their Sam Brown belts, and their glitter of bright work— shields, buttons, buckles, the row of cartridges, and the pistols swinging from their sides.

At the emergency room door, a young woman, Alice Fall, stood alert. She ran to meet me.

Alice Fall had been the type of attractive ash blonde that fades quickly under stress and sorrow, of which she had had her share. Tonight, she was distraught.

"O Doctor, save him, save him!" she cried.

"Who is it? What has happened?" I asked.

"It's Homer. He's been shot."

"For heaven's sake!" I exclaimed. "Why can't he stay out of trouble? He just left here."

I walked into the emergency room. Homer Fall lay on the operating table. Anxiously he looked toward the door; I could see his relief when he recognized me. We had been through some tight places together.

Homer was a heavyset, full-bodied man of thirty-five years. His neck was short and thick, his arms strong. His height—well, it could be anything he cared to make it—as I will explain later.

His pulse was weak. He was pale, perspiring, and breathing with difficulty. In spite of all this, to my experienced eye he did not appear to be mortally wounded. He was cold but from the night rather than from that internal chill I had seen so often. I was told that he had seemed much worse at first and that his condition had steadily improved.

There was a bullet wound to the left of the sternum, just above the heart, and another near the middle of the right chest. We turned him over but there was no wound of exit. There were signs of a considerable amount of blood in the right thoracic cavity. This lung had collapsed. An x-ray film showed two steel-jacketed bullets lodged in the muscles of the back, far out on the right side. Just how the bullet that had entered his left side, had threaded its way through the mediastinum—that packet containing the great vessels, vital nerves, the trachea, and esophagus—without injuring some of those important structures was hard to comprehend but apparently it had done so.

As Homer continued to improve under conservative treatment, I decided against any major operative procedure unless some untoward symptom should develop.

The Getaway

Mrs. Fall was in a highly nervous state. Reassuring her, I promised to stay with her husband through the night and to call if there was a change for the worse. Finally, I persuaded her to take a sedative and go to bed.

Hour after hour of observation passed—anxious observation at first—during which time I visited Homer's room, administered various treatments which I thought might be of help, wandered up and down the halls, and talked to the policemen about the happenings of the night.

At last the dawn came. The patient was so much improved that I could definitely decide against a major operation. I might as well say here that he went on to an uneventful recovery.

During these hours of waiting, I recalled what I had known of Homer's former injury and his life since then.

It had been only a few months since Homer Fall had left my care. How well I remembered the day I had first seen him! Then his condition was really desperate. He had been caught in a premature explosion at a quarry. Both legs had been destroyed from the thighs down. Pieces of stone—one piece half as large as a man's fist—were embedded in his flesh. After a long and stormy siege, he recovered.

The corporation for which he had worked made a generous settlement with him. Using a part of this money, he, with much wisdom, set about providing himself with the means for making a livelihood. He had himself outfitted with two artificial legs, which, although swung from shoulder straps, served to carry him around with a fair degree of stability. He bought acreage some distance from the city. Upon this property he built a filling station, and in the wooded area behind this he built a small, attractive, and well-appointed home. Finally, he ordered and received delivery on a new car. After all this there was still a goodly sum of money remaining— money he planned to keep for an emergency or some future investment.

Homer's business prospered based on his amiable disposition, his eagerness to oblige, and the local motorists' knowledge of his accident. He seemed in a fair way to enjoy a useful and a happy life when the new blow fell.

It was from the police sergeant that I now heard the following amazing story, most of which had been told to him by Mrs. Fall.

Near midnight Homer and his wife were awakened by a loud "Hello!" from their front yard. When Homer answered, a man said that he had run out of gasoline and asked that someone come to the station to fill his tank. Mrs. Fall helped her husband dress and followed him to the door to assist him with his coat.

When Homer opened the door, two men with leveled pistols ordered him to turn over to them the rather large amount of money they said they knew he had secreted in the house. Homer, himself a powerful man, attempted to close the door against them. Two shots rang out. Homer fell just within the door. One bandit went through Homer's pockets, taking his wallet and car keys. The other pointed his pistol at Mrs. Fall and on threat of instant death demanded that she produce the money.

She led the way to a closet and, having removed a loose board behind some clothes, gave all that was left of her husband's settlement into the bandit's hands. Almost immediately she heard the car start in the garage some distance from the house. Quickly glancing into the folder to see that the money was there, the remaining robber, brandishing his gun and threatening to kill her if she turned in an alarm, stepped over Homer as he lay gasping in the doorway and ran to the garage.

Mrs. Fall hastily called the police station for help. As she turned from the telephone, she heard a commotion in the garage, the roar of the car's motor and then the slamming of the car door. She glanced out the window. This was the act that probably saved her life. In the light streaming from the garage, she saw, not the car, but the two bandits rush out and heard their running feet on the cement walk as they raced for the house. Swiftly, she opened the kitchen door and slipped out into the black night and still blacker woods.

She was not a moment too soon. From her stand she saw lights go on in all the windows, saw through the windows the forms of the men, heard the slamming of doors and the noise of overturned furniture as they searched the house.

Out of the kitchen door came the men. Around and around the house and back to the garage they dashed. She heard the motor roar again. Again, the car door slammed.

Now, back to the house they came. They seized Homer and half-carrying, half-dragging him started toward the garage. He lay limp and heavy in their arms. They stopped and then dropped him. Again, they ran through the house and out and around it and now into the woods. They called Mrs. Fall by name, threatening her with death if she did not come out of her hiding and promising not to harm her if she did.

Cursing now and calling her dreadful names, they came close to her. She stood motionless behind a tree and held her breath. Down the drive they raced to the filling station and then to the road. As if hoping for a car that they could stop, they waited for a brief time. No car came. Now, shrieking in an utter frenzy of rage, frustration and fear, they ran back and into the garage.

With their sirens screaming, police cars raced down the road, swept into the drive, and stopped. Their spotlights showed the bandits charging from the garage, blazing guns in their hands. There were the scattered, answering shots as the officers spread out and then the rattle of a riot gun. The robbers fell.

Cautiously, weapons in hand, the officers approached the brilliant oval their spotlight marked out. There was no movement. The gunmen were dead.

It was a terrified, trembling figure that called to the officers and advanced from the woods to tell her story.

The money was found in the pocket of one of the slain men.

The officers brought Homer and his wife to the hospital.

"Why did the robbers mill around like that?" I asked. "What were they searching for? Why didn't they leave?"

"We can't figure it out," said the sergeant. "The robbery seemed carefully planned. The men walked in. They evidently expected to make their getaway in Homer's car. Why they didn't drive off is beyond me."

In the sick room, a little later, I repeated my question to Homer. He laughed outright, for all the pain it caused him.

"They couldn't drive my car," he said. "I have no legs. The controls were made especially for me."

The Wonder Drug

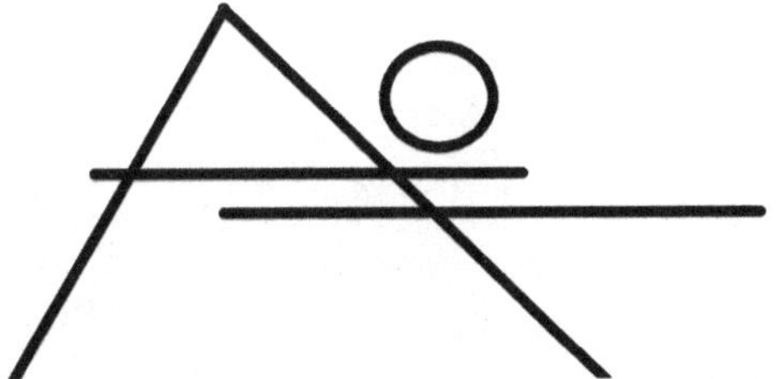

The Wonder Drug

"They tell me Dr. Ben is out of town and won't be back until tomorrow. Father is bad today and we can't wait. Will you come to see him?" Miss Sidell telephoned one winter afternoon.

"What is the matter?" I asked.

"He is restless and confused. He thinks it is raining on him," she replied.

"Is that all that's the matter? Has he gotten wet?"

"No, it hasn't been raining, he just thinks it has. Will you come?"

"Yes," I said. "It will be the early part of the night before I can get there, but I will come."

Dr. Ben White, my young associate, had told me about Miss Sidell and her father.

"He is a veteran of the Civil War and over ninety-six years of age. His daughter is nearly as old as he is," Dr. Ben had said. "There are just the two of them. They scrape along on his pension. Every time the old man gets a little ill his daughter nearly has a fit. I don't know whether all of her concern is for her dad or whether some of it is because she wouldn't know what to do without his pension. When I give the old man medicine, she will taste it and, if she doesn't fancy it, she won't give it to him."

Dark was just settling in when I finished my work at the hospital and began to think about preparations for my call.

"What should I give him?" I asked myself. He probably needs only to be reassured. Perhaps I should give him some sedative. It will have to be something mild. Old folks don't stand medicine well. The Sidells certainly have no money to spend on drugs he doesn't really need. I can probably find something here that will do. I can always telephone the pharmacy if there is anything really wrong.

These were the thoughts that passed through my mind as I made my way to the drawers where samples of drugs were kept. Every mail and every visit from a drug salesman brought in more samples. The pharmaceutical manufacturers, with their laboratories and their great staffs of research men, were forever mixing and blending drugs, old and new, into some palatable and attractive formula for which great claims would be made. A trade name would be given the mixture—a name which, as likely as not, would be one formed of some grouping of letters from the manufacturer's name rather than one chosen to give a hint of the bottle's contents. New ones superseded many of these formulas before we had a real chance to try the old.

"Something really good this time," the salesman would say. Some of these samples we gave to our patients to try. Others we set aside into two large drawers with the idea that a need for them might arise.

I rummaged through the drawers and picked up and read the formulas on the labels of bottle after bottle. Some were for whooping cough, some for the various diseases of women. There were laxatives, antiseptics, and tonics. At last, I came to a four-ounce bottle of some thin, reddish liquid. I didn't bother to look at the trade name or the name of the manufacturer. I glanced at the formula. It contained a mixture of drugs, among them a mild sedative—I have forgotten just which one.

This will do, I thought. The other drugs in the formula might build him up a little. At least they won't hurt him. I read the directions, "A teaspoonful every four or six hours." I carried the bottle to the sink, washed off the old label, stuck a piece of adhesive on the bottle, and upon this wrote the directions. I then put the bottle in my pocket.

The address given was one of the older but no longer fashionable streets of the city. Looking for the number, I drove along until I came to a small house built, along with several others, in front of an old mansion. I parked my car. It was only a few steps to the porch. Miss Sidell met me at the door and ushered me into the almost bare front room of their little home.

She seemed quite concerned as she said, "Father hasn't been at all well lately. He couldn't sleep last night. He thinks he is back in the Army. All day he has complained of the rain."

I asked her several questions but could bring out no symptoms for which age alone would not account.

"He is getting so forgetful and confused," she said. "At times I think he knows me, but I can never be sure."

She opened a door. As I looked into the room, my eyes fell upon a large, battered dishpan in the center of the bare floor. There was no water in it, none around it. The ceiling was dry.

"I put it there to humor him about the rain," she said.

Upon a small iron bed in the far corner of the room lay a feeble old man—so feeble that his bushy white eyebrows and chin whiskers seemed the most substantial things about him.

He was as shriveled as an apple that has clung to its tree all winter. A patchwork quilt, worn but clean, covered him.

His daughter told him who I was. I walked over and, taking a small straight chair, sat down by his bed and looked into what had once been a handsome face—a face now lined and wasted with the years. The eyes he turned to me with some apprehension showed those white arcs of the aged in their faded irises. The lower lids, drooping, allowed some of their lining to show. The skin of the face was thin—almost translucent.

"I have come to try to help you," I said. "Tell me the trouble."

"It's the rain," he replied. "I am so tired of it."

"Let me see about you first, and then I will attend to that," I told him.

With tremulous and clumsy hands, he tried to help me unbutton his bed jacket. He was extremely thin. I felt the flesh of his arms. It was so soft and flabby as to be almost nonexistent. With the stethoscope I listened to his breathing and to the soft beat of his heart.

The muscles of his heart are as flabby as the muscles of his arms, I thought. I finished the examination. The symptoms must have been caused by age alone. There was nothing else.

I took the bottle from my pocket.

"Bring me a spoon and a little water," I said to the daughter.

"But the rain?" queried the old man as I handed the glass to him.

"Take this and go to sleep," I told him. "The rain will stop. It will be a sunny day tomorrow."

It wasn't long before he turned on his side and, drawing up his knees, one slightly higher than the other, closed his eyes and drifted off into forgetfulness. What little flesh he had sagged downward. In all, he was but an armful of the once-powerful man.

In the outline of his form there was no suggestion of motion, no promise for the future. He had long since been pressed dry of everything this world could use. He was now weary with that weariness that water and food and rest cannot ease, for there was no thirst, no hunger, and rest itself had become unbearable.

I still sat by his bed. The old man was not the only one to see visions that night. As I gazed at him, I thought of him as he must have been—a rosy-cheeked little boy playing on the greensward as his parents watched, a lover in May with the garlands he had picked, a soldier. I saw the marching ranks of ten thousand men, their banners floating in the sky. I looked at the end of his life as it must have seemed to him that night—a great barren, desolate plain where his comrades had camped and then marched on, leaving one figure, a rear guard, who now drew his tattered cape about him against the rain, spread his thin, frail hands to the smoldering embers of the bivouac's last fire, and awaited its extinction that he might join them.

He was sleeping quietly now and comfortably. I arose and, on tiptoe, slipped from the room.

At the front door the old man's daughter said, "Thank you for coming, Doctor. What do I owe you?"

"Nothing," I replied. "Let me know how he gets along."

She thanked me again as I pulled on my coat and gloves.

"Dr. Ben also has been very kind," she told me as I left.

I stayed longer than I realized, I said to myself, for a light film of snow now covered the ground. The snow had ceased, however, and the air was clear.

I walked to the car, pulled off my right glove, and began to feel in my pockets for the key. I did not find it immediately, and, as I felt first in one pocket and then in another, I chanced to turn somewhat. A movement seen with the corner of my eye caused me to look toward the house, not twenty feet away.

Through the curtainless window I saw Miss Sidell standing in full light, which I now observed came from two electric bulbs, one on each side of the chimney breast above the mantel. She was holding the bottle of medicine I had given her up against a bulb and with ludicrous intensity was watching the light shine through. She slowly turned the bottle in her hand. She shook it, tipped it upside down, righted it, pulled the cork from it, and touched the cork to her tongue. I could see her slowly licking and sucking her lips as if giving careful consideration to the taste. She replaced the cork and again held the bottle to the light.

She is a good one if she finds out what that is, I thought. I don't know myself.

By this time, I had found the key and, after unlocking my car, climbed in and drove away.

Several days later Miss Sidell telephoned, asking that I send some more of the medicine.

"How is your father?" I asked. "Did the medicine stop the rain?"

"Yes, it did, Doctor, but he needs it again," she said. "It is the best medicine my father has ever had. He felt better while taking it than he had felt in years."

"I have no more of that," I said in some confusion, trying in vain to remember what it was. "I will telephone the drugstore to send him something that will help."

"Tell them to send a bottle of the same kind," she said. "That is what he wants."

"They don't have it," I replied.

"Can't they order it for him?"

"No."

"Why not?"

"Uh . . . there just isn't any more," I said. "That was all there was."

There was a long pause at the other end of the line, and then, "Well, ask Dr. Ben to come."

The Boy and the Bauble

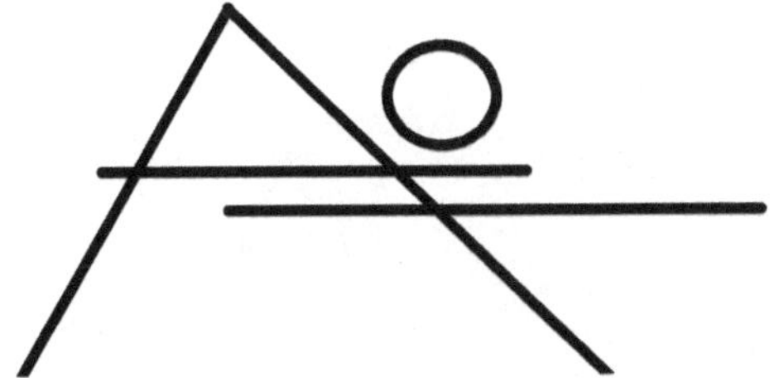

The Boy and the Bauble

Brake stick in hand, Henry Curtis trod the running board of a moving boxcar. It went to his head like wine.

"This is railroading!" he cried in exultation, waving his stick as he rolled past the old switchman standing at the entrance to the track his car was entering.

Henry had been assigned to a crew of men engaged in switching. They were breaking up a freight train which had come into the terminal and were switching its cars onto the various yard tracks where trains were being assembled—trains that could carry these cars to their various destinations.

From the top of his car, Henry's eyes swept the freight yard with its maze of gleaming rails, its creeping and standing locomotives and cars. He looked beyond to a long train pulling into the yard. It was for all the world like the toy yard in his own room at home, only a million times greater. A light rain had fallen and passed. The air and the world seemed dazzlingly bright to him.

Henry's age was twenty-one years and one day, and this was his second day at his new job. He was in size a man but still boyish in heart and appearance with pink cheeks, light brown hair, and the clear, free eye of the adventurer. He was the lover of physical toil for its own sake and for its achievement rather than for the money it brought, the lover of power and its control.

His blue overalls were new, fresh, unsullied. A red bandanna fluttered at his neck. The long bill of his blue and white cap, set jauntily upward, matched the smile that showed his even, white teeth. In boyish pride, he glanced down at his new yellow and white cloth gloves with their wide cuffs. Through the soles of his new shoes—shoes too new, stiff, and thick for his perilous stand—he felt the vibrations, the swell and fall of the great mass of the car now rolling beneath his own feet. The singing of the flange on the rails was music to his ears. This was the life—what he had always wanted! Now it was the yard, soon it would be the open road, and then the world beyond.

The switchmen, after bringing their cars to a stop, usually walked back, caught, and climbed upon the next ones as they were cut from the train. Now, however, the train had come to a switch deep within the maze and Henry, having just brought his cars to a stop close to this point, ran to catch the train for the ride back. Now he was on the train once more as it moved into the main lead for room to kick the next cars into their sidings.

He felt the speed of the cars lessen. He glanced toward the cab at the engineer he admired and respected so much. The locomotive stopped. A heavy blow of steel on steel, repeated again and again, passed from car to car like a palpable chain of sound as the slack ran through. There was a jerk as his own car came to a rest—a jerk that caused his feet to slide on the wet boards of the narrow walk. As inexperienced as he was, he thought nothing of this.

Now he glanced at the man standing at the switch of the track his own car was to take. Henry saw him stoop and throw the heavy, weighted bar and step upon it to press it home. He swung his hand in a signal for the return. Again, Henry felt the movement of the train with its great momentum, the swelling speed for the final push. He saw the yard conductor, list of car numbers in hand, step forward from his station to cut the cars he rode from the others.

Henry alone controlled them now. It seemed as if he soared. He waved to the switchman as he passed. Now he stood at the brake wheel. Now he spun it in his hands. Now he seized its rim to tighten it. The cars slackened their speed somewhat but still rapidly rolled on. He had miscalculated their speed and had been late in tightening the brake. Perhaps the push was greater than usual, perhaps the number of cars greater. They were moving fast, too fast to strike the other cars on the track without damage. He ineptly took his left hand from the brake wheel. Quickly, he inserted the stick between the radials of the wheel and, grasping it with both hands, gave a mighty tug. His feet shot from under him. Clutching wildly at the empty air, he plunged headfirst, downward between the rolling cars. As he fell, he struggled desperately to catch the cutoff rod. Missing it he fell across the rail. Instantly he seized a rod above. The gloved fingers of his right hand, jammed between the rod and the car, dragged him before the wheels as he struggled to avoid them. A few seconds more and the cars would bump and stop. A fold of his overalls became caught within the nip of the flange, arresting his movement. Seized in that giant vise, he was borne down by those ponderous wheels as they passed over both thighs, crushing and holding them to the rail. At one and the same time, the wheels, rolling onward, carrying the truck and car in which his hand had become engaged, tore his right arm from his body.

Two switchmen, walking back from their cars, saw the accident and ran to Henry. One stayed with him, while the other spread the alarm and summoned an ambulance.

Grim-faced attendants brought his stretcher into the operating room. His face was shrunken, waxen, pallid with the pallor of death, and covered with cold, clammy perspiration. His eyes were deep in their sockets. Their pupils were widely dilated, giving their glassy stare a weird and unearthly look. His features were pinched, his lips cyanotic and bloodless. His respiration, except for the occasional half gasp of air hunger, was reduced to the minimum. I put my finger over the artery that coursed up his temple. There was no pulse.

He looked up at me, as would some mortally stricken animal. There was no moan or cry of pain. This injury was too deep for that. There was no inquiry as to whether or not he would survive. He knew. This one misstep, one instant of inattention, was to be his last. There would be for him no second chance.

"Put him on the table," I said.

The attendants held back for an instant as if they would shrink from uncovering him. I myself turned back the spread and blankets from a dark, torn, and twisted mass, all coated with clotted blood, coal dust, and cinders.

"Quick! Put him on the table," I ordered.

Compassionate arms were now about his body, lifting him. Others caught up and supported his legs, which, held to him by naught but a tattered and frayed cloth, dropped downward as he was moved.

I tilted the table to bring his head much lower than his body so that what little blood remained would run by gravity to his brain.

With bandage, shears, and knives; we set about cutting his clothes from him. The thick, twisted seams were difficult to cut. We hastened with all possible speed. Some straps were unbuckled, some cut. We rolled and lifted him so that his clothes could be pulled from beneath him. Then, the grimy, terrible mass—sodden, blackened, and torn clothes; legs and feet with the shoes still on—all crushed and mangled—came away together in one great, gruesome armful and was piled to one side. I looked down upon that ghastly and pathetic ruin.

It seemed no longer a man. His body was cold, pallid, dying, oozing drops of cold and clammy perspiration at every pore. He was not bleeding now; he was exsanguinated.

The nurses rapidly sponged him with warm water and then began to dry and warm him.

In a labored, halting voice Henry spoke for the first and only time.

"Doctor, did it hurt my watch?"

I glanced at his face and perceived the darkening shadow upon it. His eyes turned to his clothes.

"See," I told a nurse, "and quickly."

Two nurses poked and pulled at the grimy mess with long tongs, trying to untangle it. Henry, using his remaining strength, raised himself and rolled slightly, the better to follow the search. In his eagerness to see the watch, he had forgotten all else. His eyes followed the ends of the tongs as they pulled and dragged his clothes this way and that. Presently, one of the nurses found it.

"No," she said, "it is all right. It is still running," and, wiping the dark blood from it, she stepped forward and dangled it before his eyes.

Henry narrowly looked at the watch. It was a beautiful watch, large, a railroad watch of bright yellow gold hanging by its golden chain. Satisfied, he sank back. A faint smile came to his face, he closed his eyes, and death, that balm of the hopeless, came to him.

As I stood and looked at that terrible scene, I thought of the irrevocable nature of so many of our actions, the one misstep that makes the difference between sunny life with its promise and black death. This boy today, another tomorrow! When will it be our own time to come to that Golgotha, and of what form will its torment be? "For none can tell to what red Hell / His sightless soul may stray."[2]

I thought of these things, but most of all I thought of the vanity of possessions. I tried yet failed to understand the mentality and the activating force behind an interest in a material possession, a bauble, at a time when a kingdom would be so much dross—a vain and empty thing.

It was many a year later that a tall, white-haired man, a builder so he said, came to me. His name meant nothing to me at first.

---

2. Oscar Wilde, "The Ballad of Reading Gao," in *The Top 500 Poems*, ed. William Harmon (New York: Columbia University Press, 1992), 815, lines 23-24.

After I had examined him and had given him my advice, he arose as if to go, stood silently, and then said, "Doctor, I had a son once, an only son. You were with him when he died. His name was Henry Curtis. Do you remember him?"

"Yes," I replied. "I remember him very well."

"He was a good boy," Mr. Curtis said. "Only once did he ever insist on doing a thing that I asked him not to do. I begged him to stay in school and give up the idea of a job on the railroad, but that was what he wanted, what he had looked forward to all his life. He wouldn't have been satisfied with anything else. It had to be, but I can never get him out of my mind. To see or to hear a train is to live it over again. For a long time, I couldn't speak of him. Many a time I wanted to come and see you, to thank you, to talk of Henry but I could not."

"Sit down," I said to him, putting my hand on his shoulder. "Sit down and tell me about him. It will help you. It will help us both."

He told me of Henry's first ride on a train, of his play at running one, of the toy trains he had assembled at home, of how he had looked forward to the time when he would be old enough to take a job on the railroad, of how he thought his entry into this job was a fitting way to celebrate his birthday, and of what he had said about his work that first and only night that he had lived to speak of it.

"You might think it strange," the father said, "but I don't. I have seen little boys preaching to their playmates. I have seen born aviators. I know a boy who played at being a doctor until he became one. My boy was a railroader. He would have made a good one."

Mr. Curtis had come to the end of his story. I sat in quietness, not replying at once.

"Do you really remember him?" he asked suddenly. "Are you sure you remember my boy?"

"Yes, I remember him," I replied. "I was thinking of his watch. His only concern seemed to be for its safety. The only words he spoke were to ask if it had been injured."

The father took from his pocket a watch of bright yellow gold.

"This is the watch," he said.

"I have often thought of it," I began, my eyes upon it. "All railroad men prize their watches. To many it is their most cherished possession—valuable, often beautiful, a bright spot no matter how grimy their work . . . but why Henry . . . at such a time . . . I suppose though . . . a boy . . ."

"No, Doctor," said the father, "it wasn't that. This was my watch. Henry borrowed it from me and gave his word that no harm would come to it."

An Uncompleted Call

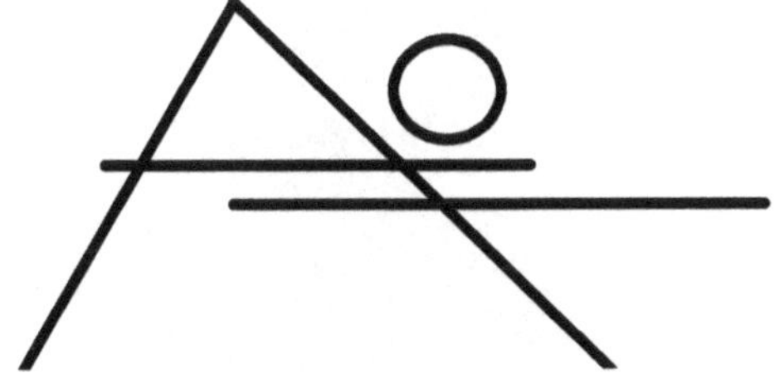

An Uncompleted Call

"Mr. Jessup is on the phone," said my secretary to me one morning. "He wanted you to come to his house right away and when I told him you couldn't, he insisted upon talking to you."

I took up the receiver. "This makes four times I have called for you," said a rasping, acrid voice, "and each time the girl in your office has given me some cock-and-bull story about how busy you are. What's the matter? I paid you, didn't I?"

"I don't do General Practice," I reminded him. "I don't make any outside calls unless it is an emergency."

"How do you know this is not an emergency?" he demanded. "I want you to come and see."

I held back for a moment and then replied, "Let my secretary give you an appointment here at the hospital. It will only be a day or two before I can see you. I couldn't examine you properly at your home. All my instruments and any help I might need are here."

"I have no way of coming," Mr. Jessup replied.

"You could call a taxi," I suggested.

"No, I want you to come here," he said with mounting anger. "Are you coming or not?"

"I am due in the operating room in a few minutes," I replied. "I can't come. Who is your regular physician?"

An explosion of fury burst in my ear and then came the bang and clatter as he slammed down his receiver.

A year before, I had operated upon him for a minor ailment. He got along very well but not to hear him tell it. As a patient in the hospital, he had been most exacting with me and most willful and notionate in accepting treatment. Try as they might, the nurses could do nothing to please him. Since that time, he had been to see me, had called and had written—all to blame me for everything bad that had ever happened to him.

When the morning's surgery was over and I had returned to my desk, I found Mr. Jessup's name on the list of those who had called and left their number.

I will tell him that where mutual respect and confidence are disturbed, a doctor should not attempt to treat a patient. I prompted myself to say that it would be much better for both of us if he would call another doctor. As I turned to the telephone it occurred to me that I might have no opportunity to say my speech. He just wants to haul me over the coals again. Well, it is better to get it over and done with. I called his number.

With his very first words my resentment began to drain away. His voice was soft, almost seductive.

"I want to apologize to you, Doctor," he began. "I can't get out now and was fretted for a moment. Please don't be angry with an old man. I am sick and despondent. I don't want anyone else. I want you and am willing to wait. It is only a few blocks off your way as you go home. Please forgive me—and come."

"It's all right. Let's forget it," I told him and then added, "I will be glad to see you if you are really sick and really want me, but why can't you come here like everyone else? What is the matter?"

There was a long pause. "I can't tell you very well over the phone," was the reply when it finally came. "Let me tell you when you get here. Any time will do just so it is before dark. I . . . I go to bed early."

Reluctantly, but to do my share of the peacemaking, I promised to make the call.

"Let me think for a minute," I told him and then, "Look for me at five o'clock."

Later that afternoon I left my work—work that would still keep me into the night—and in a somewhat disgruntled frame of mind started the drive to his house.

I promised myself not to go," I said aloud, "and here I am, getting into it again."

Mr. Jessup was a dried-up, little old man. No one here knew anything of his early life. He had come to the city a few years before and bought a small, isolated house on a side street. He soon acquired a reputation as being eccentric and overbearing. For a while he ran an advertisement in the local paper stating that he had money with which to make small loans secured by chattel mortgages. Having made a number of such loans, Mr. Jessup retired into his house. There, like a spider, he lay in wait, emerging from time to time to collect his interest or to prey on some defaulting victim who had become entangled in his web. He lived alone. He had no family, no friends— certainly none locally. He belonged to no church, no club. Few, I had been told, had ever seen inside his house. It seemed always shut up. As time passed, Mr. Jessup refused all proffers of friendship and left his house less and less often, until finally he became almost a recluse.

What devilish schemes drift through that crafty mind as day after day he sits and broods? I wondered, half aloud.

Presently, I came within sight of his smoke-stained, gray house. It was a small, one-story structure, set upon the very crest of the hill. Across its front was a porch draped with some heavy-leafed vine. The large lot surrounding the house was devoid of vegetation.

Now, the house was out of view. I had driven into the deep cut where the road ran through the top of the hill. I stopped my car. All I could see was a high, red clay bank and its flight of steep, wooden steps. As I climbed these, I glanced along a walk which thirty feet away, came to two or three steps and an opening in the vines.

I must have looked down, my mind must have wandered for a moment. I had walked the length of the path and had put my foot upon the first step when suddenly I was impelled to look up. I froze. Not more than a yard away from my face, a gigantic savage head blocked my way. The details I saw were long, heavy, milk-white fangs laid bare by curling red lips; and then, looking beyond, I gazed into a pair of cold, appraising eyes that glared into my own. I felt more than saw that it was some great dog—but what a dog! No nightmare could have dreamed up such a beast. As he stood upon the porch, his great out-thrust head was level with my own.

What should I do? After consideration I spoke very gently and quietly to him. His eyes narrowed and became fiercer. I thought of ordering him to one side.

This might work and again it might not, I thought. He was too close, too powerful for me to correct an error once it was made. No, it would take someone more dominant, someone endowed with more temerity than was I, to attempt that.

I momentarily expected Mr. Jessup and thought of calling for him but feared the slightest movement or sound might be enough to invoke a furious attack. I glanced toward the nearest window. It was closed and heavily curtained. I felt the dog's hot breath. Instantly, my eyes jerked back to the beast. He was edging closer. There was no sound from the house; I dared not look again. The thought of retreat came to me.

No, I won't be chased off by a dog not even this one, I resolved.

This firm decision steadied me somewhat, and I remembered that by looking an animal straight in the eye he could be cowed. Summoning all the feeling of command which for the moment was at my disposal, I looked sternly into those great eyes.

My attempt to stare him down but fanned his anger. His eyes now glowed like coals of fire when the breath is blown upon them. The coarse, stiff, tawny bristles on the back of his neck lifted. His mouth jerked open in a sudden, savage snarl. I felt my hat move slightly as my own hair rose. His lips now tightened and lifted. He drew them sharply back, showing the full length of his massive teeth. His mouth opened yet wider and I looked into a red, cavernous throat and at giant jaws that could take my head into their lock and crush it as easily as they could crush a beef hock and that like an eggshell. There was now a low, harsh, guttural sound deep in his chest.

Still, I attempted to stare him down; but as he slowly rocked forward on his legs, stretching his neck yet farther, and bringing his snarling, dripping nose and fangs closer and closer—within inches of my face—I was the one to give ground. As I slowly drew back, he continued to rock forward on his legs and stretch his neck toward me. I eased myself backward, my eyes fixed upon his. He did not follow. Back I stepped, still slowly back, until I came to the steps leading to the sidewalk. With the same slow movement, I backed down until the great dog and the house were lost from view. Quickly, I opened the door of my car and sprang into its safety.

I was trembling now that the strange encounter was over. Along with my relief came a feeling of humiliation that I, a superior being far up on the evolutionary scale, could have been scared out of countenance and almost out of my wits by a dog. It didn't help much to consider that he was too low on the scale to realize how obnoxious he had made himself, too ignorant to realize the importance of my visit, and too far beneath me in worth to be a respecter of persons. No, there was nothing personal in his manner, I decided. To him, a college professor was not as important as a side of beef.

Then, as I sat and considered the animal's great strength and acuteness of his facilities, I began to wonder whether, after all, evolution had been so kind to me. I can claim superiority if I want to, I thought, but certainly by the dog's standard that is far from true. He knows who is the best man—the best dog I mean. He knows that I am no match for him, that his teeth are better than mine.

It occurred to me that Don Quixote under somewhat similar circumstances stood his ground, but then he was encased in a suit of armor with a shield in one hand and a sword in the other. Not only that, his lion was a whelp in comparison to this beast.

Having reached some degree of composure, I blew my horn and waited. There was no response.

That's strange, I thought. Why doesn't Mr. Jessup come? And then perhaps he can't hear the horn, perhaps the bank deflects the sound. Again, I blew the horn, this time long and loud, and again waited. Mr. Jessup knew that I was coming at five o'clock. He should have kept the dog in the house.

Another thought, a most disquieting one, suddenly crowded forward. Did he want to hear my horn?

My mind drifted back over the details of my adventure. It came to a point and stopped. In that one fleeting glance which I had taken, an image in the window had indelibly fixed itself upon my retina. At the time I had been too preoccupied with the dog to take it all in, but now I could see it with startling clarity. The curtain stood a little out from the side of the window, and through that opening, someone peeped at me.

I started my car and drove on to join other players, amid other drops, on this eternal stage.

Amends with a Vengeance

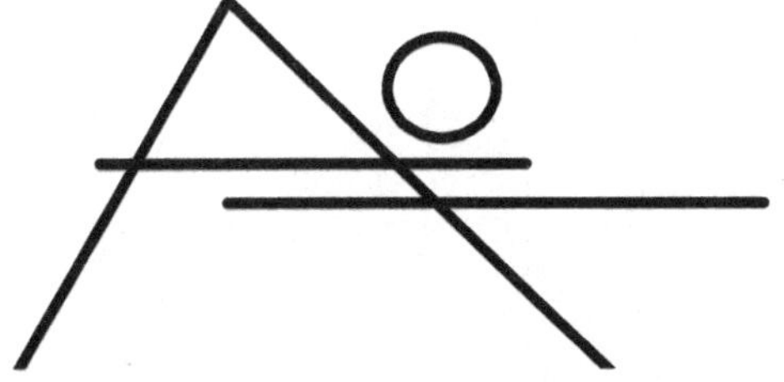

Amends with a Vengeance

Blow, blow, thou winter wind,
Thou art not so unkind
As man's ingratitude.
Shakespeare

Thus, wrote the Bard of Avon, stung to the quick.

The ingratitude of which he speaks—that is, the forgetfulness of favors done for others—never troubled me. I myself have been all too derelict in this respect to be exacting of others. I have made many mistakes in my time—left the kind, helpful word unsaid, withheld my hand when I might have aided—still inexcusable even when from shyness and reserve. Praise and even thanks have always brought to me a sense of uneasiness by reminding me of all those times when I have failed. All in all, I have been happy—I might say almost anxious—to let both the good and the bad of my past go along together and be forgotten.

There is another type of ingratitude, one that is extremely rare, and it is well that it is, for a little of it goes a long way. I speak of an active attempt to injure a benefactor, an attempt made by one who has been befriended and cared for with no thought or prospect of remuneration.

Such an action by one of my former patients came to my attention and nettled me once. After I had spoken to the man about it, however, and saw what his true feelings were, I took this for a lesson and forever afterwards was willing to let this kind of ingratitude pass with the others. I realized that, after all, it was only thoughtlessness on his part. Indeed, he was deeply concerned at the success of his one-man campaign against me. Furthermore, he did something about it. He put his wits to work to save me from disaster and came up with a most ingenuous and surprising solution. Just how this solution might appeal to the other doctor concerned, I shall leave to your imagination.

Gib Parks was more of a mountaineer than he was a mill worker. He owned a mountain cove and a boundary of rough land running up the slope to join the government's game preserve. Here he lived in a small two-room house by the roadside. Hunting and fishing together with the cutting of a little cordwood had been, or at least had appeared to be, his main occupation for most of his life—until the revenue officers caught him red-handed at a blockade still.

After serving a term in the penitentiary, he returned home and secured work as a laborer in a great mill several miles from his home. The daily drive back and forth in his jalopy, the labor, and the confining life at the mill must have been a sore trial for one who had killed as many bears as had he, for one who had whipped the trout streams since childhood; but evidently the even more irksome confinement he had undergone had made a believer out of him, so he stuck to his job. His real nature was not changed, however. The love of the mountains was still in his blood, perhaps that morning a little mountain dew as well in the light of what happened.

While others at the mill had taken their vacations in the summertime, Gib had saved his for the fall. Now he was off for a week. He and a number of his cronies had organized a bear hunt and were out in the frozen night. Two men were with the dogs, the rest were scattered out at their various stands to intercept the bear as he was driven past.

From his stand in the mountain gap at the government line, Gib heard the dogs strike the trail. Their cry was music to his ears. He could pick out and identify the bark of each dog.

That's old Lead, he thought, my dog, the best in the pack. That deep voice is Jowler's.

He listened to the lighter cry of the youngsters. The dogs circled the cove and came across the slope of the mountain far below him. Now they were beyond the ridge and the sound of the hunt was faint. Then he heard its sound increase. All at once there was a savage swell in the bark of the dogs and, as he told me later, he knew they had sighted the bear. There came the rush down the mountainside as bear and pack, like a runaway team and wagon, swept through a cutover area with its heavy brush and undergrowth. Now the outcry told Gib the dogs were upon the bear's heels. Next the snarling, savage, yelping pack was upon him, all over him. Gib heard the cry of a hound as it received its mortal blow and the mingled outcries of the beasts as the furious, tangling mass of bear and dogs rolled over and over, breaking down saplings, crushing and uprooting the bushes. Now the bear was on his feet, the pack upon his heels, all of them fighting as they came. Now they were in the clear and making straight for the gap. Gib cocked his gun and stood tense, in readiness. They veered off and passed below him. He lowered the muzzle of his gun and strained his eyes in an attempt to catch a glimpse of them in the first, faint light of dawn. There was a loud report from his high-powered rifle, and Gib felt a stinging pain in his right foot.

A little later, a tall, lanky man of thirty-eight years was admitted to my service at the hospital. I pulled out an old shirt that had been wadded through a large hole in the sole of his shoe and cut the shoe off. On the upper surface of the arch of the foot was a small wound of entry. Within the foot the bullet had spread out and, carrying fragments of the bone with it, had blown a wide crater in the plantar surface. It was an ugly wound. Several tendons had been injured, one destroyed.

To Gib the wound seemed but a passing incident. "Cut the foot off if you think it ought to go, Doc," he said.

"Oh no," I told him. "It will take a long time for it to get well, but it will be worth it. It's a lot better than any you can buy in the store."

I cleaned the wound, did a debridement, and patched it up as well as I could.

Gib and I got along wonderfully well together; we were kindred spirits. I enjoyed hearing him talk about the forest and the life of the creatures that inhabit it. Each day I dressed his foot and the wound slowly filled in.

As time wore on, Gib became impatient. Once, he bitterly complained about the pain in the red granulating wall of the crater.

"What in the Sam Hill is the matter with it?" he wailed. "It feels like techin' a red-hot coal to your eyeball."

"It must be the end of a nerve," I said. I got a magnifying glass and searched for it in vain.

"Well, a nerve is a little art-tickle," he said, "but it sure hurts big enough."

I ended this trouble by injecting Novocain and cauterizing the area.

Amends with a Vengeance

Several times during the long treatment of his foot Gib told me that he wished I had cut it off, that it was taking too long to get well.

When the granulation had grown sufficiently, I grafted a skin flap over the raw surface and finally got him up on crutches. It wasn't long then before he was walking with very little limp. I gave him a letter saying that I thought he could resume his work at the mill.

He was now in high spirits and everything was clearing when he ran into an unexpected complication. The plant physician would not certify him for the job.

Old Dr. Evans sucked his breath through his teeth. "I want to see what's going to happen to it. Yes. . .yes. . . we'll wait awhile," he said with deceptive gentleness.

When Gib insisted and 'reckoned' that the doctor who had been treating him knew when he was all right, Dr. Evans became more severe.

"I have already told you I won't do it. You wait," he said crossly.

Gib came back to me.

"There is nothing I can do," I told him. "You know Dr. Evans. I wouldn't argue with him if I were you. If you do or if you try to go over his head, you may never get your job back. Every day you should soak your foot in warm water and rub it with . . . well, bear grease will do. Use the foot all you can, in reason, and try again in about three weeks."

He tried again but it was the same. "It's not strong enough," said Dr. Evans.

Evans was an ornery old fellow. "Sour Jim," the men called him. but not where he could hear, mind you. He had begun working at the plant when it was small, doing the physical examinations and first-aid work on a part-time basis. He was now too old for active practice and lived on the rather meager salary paid him by the mill.

I did the heavy surgery for the plant. This was the only really remunerative part of the medical work. I had obtained and kept this important work because I happened to be the choice of the men higher up, who controlled the department, rather than through any fondness Dr. Evans had for me.

The next time Gib went to the mill, the outcome was the same, and the next, and the next.

As months passed, Gib gradually got around to blaming me for all of his troubles. Presently, I began to hear some things I didn't like.

It chanced one day not long after I heard of his derogatory remarks that I had a call that took me by Gib's home. I glanced across the unkempt yard, ragged with the half-rotten stumps of forest trees cut when the house had been built. Its clay slope was littered with hounds lying around as if dead in the sun. Gib was sitting on the porch, an old, black hat pulled over his eyes, his feet on the rail. I stopped my car.

"Gib," I called. "Come down here. I want to talk to you."

He got up and with an exaggerated limp slowly came to the car. His little show made me somewhat more severe than I might have been.

"Gib," I began. "I am surprised and ashamed of you."

"Why, what's the matter?" he asked, sheepishly.

"You know what's the matter," I told him. "When you were in my hospital, I did everything I could for you, no matter how tired or how busy I was. And here you are, putting yourself out to go see my patients, trying to get them to leave me and go to young Dr. Bennett, telling everyone that he is so much better than I am."

"Why, I didn't do that," he said. "You know I wouldn't do that."

"Yes, you did," I replied with some heat. "Fred Allen wouldn't tell a lie. You made it a point to see him, and Smith Collins, and Walter Brown. All of them told me the same story. They told me to tell you what they said."

"I didn't mean no harm, Doc. I wouldn't do anything to hurt you. You and me are too good friends for that."

He put his foot up on the running board.

"How you come on anyway, Doc?" he said, in a rather hollow attempt to change the subject.

I sat and looked at him a minute. I began to soften as I saw the bid for forgiveness in his anxious face. I also saw a chance to have a little fun with him and perhaps punish him a bit at the same time.

"I am not doing any good," I replied.

"How is that?" he asked, puzzled.

"I am losing all my practice," I said, building up my exaggeration as I moved along. "These new doctors— they are young and handsome and strong. They're better prepared than I am. That's about what you said, isn't it? They are taking all my patients. That's what you wanted, wasn't it?"

"Why, when I was to see you a couple months ago, folks was sittin' all around and standin' in the yard."

"That was just a happen-so," I answered. "Not anymore! There's nobody there now—nobody!"

Seeing from his face that my shaft had found its mark, I pressed it home.

"I'm ruined, I tell you! Ruined! I don't know how I can feed my children. I just don't know what to do."

Now his jaw really dropped. He stood and looked at me in consternation—almost in tears. His fingers moved and twitched as he clutched the car door. He was in a quandary, wondering how he could right the wrong.

"Doc . . . Doc," he stammered as he sought a solution to my problem. Then his face began to clear; a nebulous idea had come to his mind.

"I'll tell you what . . . Doc," he began slowly and then, as the idea expanded, rushed to the point.

"Maybe old Evans `ul die and you can get his job at the mill."

A Water Haul

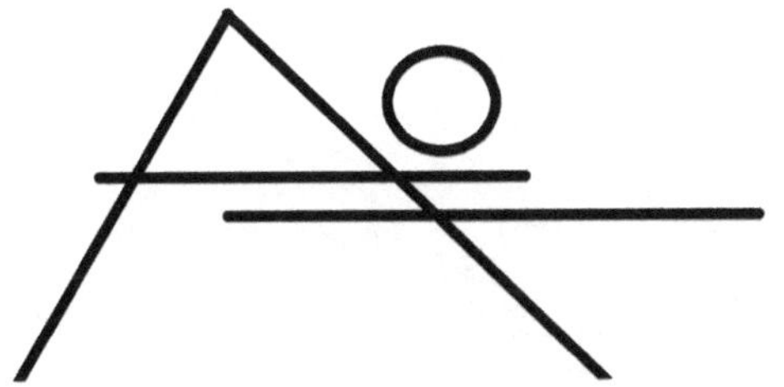

A Water Haul

"Rob-ert! Robert! Where are you?"

"What I want to know is why you didn't fix it right while you were about it!"

"Why don't you pay me?"

The first was the high, raucous voice of his wife; the second were the stern, cutting words of our efficient superintendent at the hospital; and the third was—well, a chorus joined in by just any and everyone.

Mr. Robert Jackson was, figuratively, the head of a family well known to me, my patients over several years.

He was nearing fifty years of age—a little man of the faded, sandy, freckled variety—wiry, tough, and thin. His scalp was drawn tight across his skull as if he had taken it in his two strong, bony hands and with all his strength had pulled it on and down around his ears. Below this there was skin and to spare.

He was not bald in the usual sense for everywhere over his scalp grew a sprinkling of short, faded, sandy hair. A goodly stubble of the same grew on his wrinkled face and a still better supply adorned his forearms and chest, as I noticed when, grimy and coatless, he was straining at his work.

Hurried, furtive, anxious, berated—all these words fit into the picture—I might say motion picture—of that soft-voiced little man who feverishly rushed from one job to another during those trying times of the Great Depression. Running about and around in circles, he attempted the impossible task of bringing together the loose ends that dangled from every segment at which he chanced to pause.

It is said that a husband and wife grow to resemble each other. Mr. and Mrs. Jackson did a good job of this. Except for certain minor details such as the fact that he was male and she female, she somewhat younger, disporting her faded, brittle, sandy hair on her head rather than elsewhere, they were almost identical in appearance.

They had several children. Other than their variation in size, they were all alike and all resembled their parents with the same thinness and same faded, freckled coloring.

One thing or another was forever happening to the family. In the summer a boy would fall out of a cherry tree and break his arm. Not to be outdone, the following winter one of his sisters would fall on the ice and receive a similar injury. There were rock battles and scalp wounds to be sutured. There were appendices to be removed from among the children. The wife had an operation or two. When she was a patient in the hospital, the chief thing that I remember about her stay was the large ashtray on the table beside her. No matter how often it was emptied it was always full and spilling over with foul-smelling ashes and cigarette butts, some still smoldering, piled so high that I found myself wondering where she could put the one she was smoking.

Hardly missing a stroke on her chewing gum, her high-pitched, unpleasant voice would ring out,

"Have you seen Robert? Where is that worm?"

A Water Haul

The designation was spoken half jocundly and affectionately, half as if calling attention to a fact.

Mr. Jackson was the handyman at our little hospital, not from choice of either side perhaps, but because in some way we had assumed medical care of his family; and, owing us a considerable amount, he had offered in lieu of money which he did not have, to do our work allowing us to pay one half the price of these services and apply the other half on his bill. He was more attentive to us when some member of his family had just left us than he was at other times, though I must say that at all times he did well.

Once several messages that had been left for him had gone unanswered and, since I was going to pass not far from the section in which his place of business was located, the hospital superintendent asked if I would go by to see why he had not come.

His shop was part of an old livery stable near the bank of a muddy river. Whether or not the day was unusually overcast I do not remember, but my impression was of a yawning, dark cave. There were no windows; the large, solid wooden door was open, allowing a look into its depths. My first glance disclosed the earthen floor with its piles of tools and old second-hand materials, the dust-laden cobwebs in the joists above, and the rough stones that formed the walls of that gloomy cavern.

While my eyes and mind were taking in this scene, they were at the same time leaving it and turning to another one. To the right, and well back from the door, was a soft glow and—I rubbed my eyes and looked again—yes, a young woman, a very personable one at that, sat behind the small table which served as a desk.

Jobs surely must be hard to find, I thought. She arose as I approached. She couldn't have been more than thirty-two or three. Her trim black suit, her white Peter Pan collar and white cuffs, and her fair face above all were immaculate.

The oval of light in which she stood seemed more a halo than rays from the shaded bulb above—and she some good fairy dropped amid those squalid surroundings to set things right.

"How do you do, Doctor," she greeted me pleasantly and then as I hesitated, trying to place her, continued, "I used to see you come into the bank. I worked there until it had to close. How may I help you?"

"Oh yes! Yes," I replied. "I came to see Mr. Jackson. He seems to have forgotten us."

"I am sure it isn't that. He has been busy lately and so worried too. I will ask him to call as soon as he comes back. It will be the middle of the afternoon."

"Thank you," I said and started to turn away.

"Doctor!" she stopped me. Her face was a study in seriousness as she groped for words. They came with soft intensity. "Can't you help him? Few of the people he works for can pay. He needs help as much as any of your patients. I don't have to tell you the condition he is in. He can't go on. I would help him myself, but what I have wouldn't be a start among his creditors."

"I don't know what I can do," I replied. "We are all in the same boat."

"Not quite", she corrected me.

No, we are not, I thought.

Then I said, "We had better forget the bill and pay full price for his work. That will help a little."

"Yes, a little," she repeated, disappointedly.

Mr. Jackson, on the half-run as usual, came into the hospital that afternoon. Several times in the following months I saw him there. Once I passed the superintendent talking to him in the hall. She was speaking in no uncertain terms as she told him of his unsatisfactory work. Within an hour I heard her after him again, over the telephone. There was trouble with the dishwasher drain just after he had unstopped it. I happened to see him as he answered this call. He parked his small truck well past the hospital drive. Then, slipping in the side entrance, he glanced this way and that as he attempted to avoid his nemesis. He might as well have spared himself the pains. He met her face to face.

"I can't be forever bothered with these things," she told him. "Now you stay until it is right."

Sometimes while he was at the hospital, one of his sons would come with a message of trouble at home or a list of provisions he should bring. They were now large enough to make their own money, but they would ask it of him. Sometimes he would give it to them—after quite an argument. More often than not they went away empty-handed.

"Nobody ever pays me. I am not the mint!" he had exclaimed.

Occasionally his wife would come to the hospital and each time, taking no one's word, would look about the grounds calling his name. After all these years, her harsh voice still rings in my ears.

It seemed Robert owed everyone. Bill collectors would wait in front of the hospital for him to come; others waited to bedevil him as he left.

All this seemed bad enough, but well I knew that I had witnessed only a sampling of the tormenting winds that continually swept over him.

Robert became more tremulous, thinner if possible, paler, grimmer, and more nervous.

How would it end? I did not consciously ask the question, but it was always there.

The day of reckoning came—a winter day—one of the darkest of the Great Depression. It started badly. Our superintendent told me she had been in Mr. Jackson's shop, talking to him and his secretary, when Mrs. Jackson came in.

"You should have seen her when he spoke rather sharply and said he had no money."

"What did she say?" I asked.

"She screamed he had enough to keep 'that secretary' and whacked him over the head with her umbrella."

We didn't know there was any trouble with the plumbing, but at noon Mr. Jackson came to the hospital. This time he parked his truck in the bushes behind the library. He ate his lunch in silence and then, with his wrenches, spent the afternoon in the crawlways under one of the wings.

The sun was sinking before he came out and the sheriff was waiting for him. He served Robert with a writ of assistance attaching his truck and all other property—every tool he owned. The sheriff had just left when Robert came into my office to tell the story.

"And now what?" he queried, dazed and hopeless.

"Well, you can't decide anything now," I counseled him. "Try to get some sleep. If you will wait half an hour, I can take you home."

"I feel somehow it would help me to walk," he said, and then, "I had better make sure Mary locked the shop."

I stood in the doorway and watched him limp down the walk.

It is twilight—not just for the gods; it's curtains for him, I thought. Our patients can't pay either; I can't help.

As he went, Robert leaned forward slightly and to one side. He stumbled as he walked, for all the world like some wild bird shot down, making its way into the night.

The next day when I came down from the operating room, I saw an officer standing at the end of the hall and, here and there, little groups of nurses were huddled together talking in subdued voices. There was a feeling of the unusual, of mystery, and of sadness in the air. In a bay to one side, the superintendent stood with a stranger as if she had been questioned and now could tell no more. She left him and came to me.

"Do you know where Mr. Jackson is?" she asked. "Did he spend the night at the hospital?"

"No," I replied. "Why?"

"He didn't go home last night. His son was here early this morning looking for him. They have notified the police, but they still haven't found him. Oh, I hope nothing has happened—poor soul!"

The next night I was called back to the hospital. As I drove along, I noticed a strange glow in the sky a few blocks to the west.

Our superintendent chanced to be at the hospital and as I came in, ran to meet me.

"Now guess what?" she queried.

"They have found his body," I ventured.

"No," she said. "It's about Miss Richardson. She has gone too."

"Who is Miss Richardson?" I asked.

"His secretary. I just met the woman she lives with. When I asked how Miss Richardson was taking it the woman said she packed her car that very night and left for the north to get a job. Why that night? You don't supp-o-se . . ."

"Ha! Yes I do," I muttered. "Has anyone else thought of that?" I put my fingers to my lips.

"No," she replied, as her face broke into a smile. "The whole town has gone down behind his shop. They have built great fires along the banks and are dragging the river."

The Cry in the Night

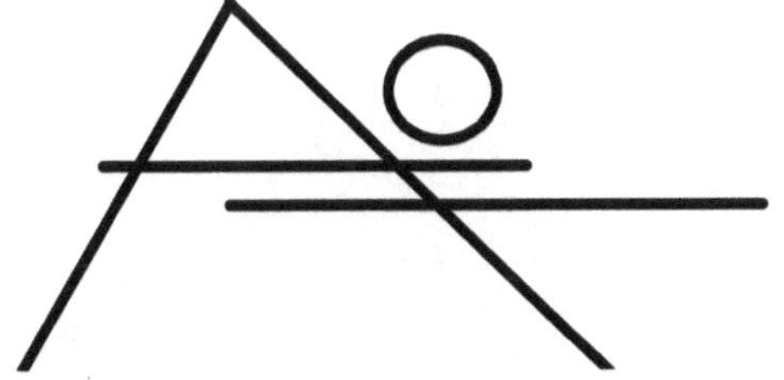

The Cry in the Night

The human body, aided by time alone, will throw off many ills. In most of the other cases, advice, the judicious use of medicine, nursing care, or an operation will restore health. Nevertheless, some illnesses forever tend to worsen and, in spite of all that can be done, end in death—an ending usually regarded as the ultimate example of the failure of a doctor's endeavors.

There is, however, a malady with which the victim's mind and body cannot cope—an illness in which the doctor's inability to aid is fraught with consequences still more terrible. It occurs when an individual, failing to see the danger inherent in a course and following what seems to him to be a well thought out and wisely planned program, is led easily and naturally, step by step, each seemingly well considered, each seemingly full of promise, until at last he is brought into a position which he finds unbearable; yet one from which there is no return. Therein follows a sickness of the soul, a sickness that cannot be palliated, one for which there is no balm, no termination—alas! No escape except in death.

It seemed but another office call when the nurse brought in the patient, introduced her, and handed me the usual forms on which was recorded her medical history.

A glance showed a small, extremely emaciated woman. Her thin face was sallow and filled with large, dark splotches. There were dark shadows and a sagging below her sunken eyes—eyes in which, as they turned to me, I could see a return of hope, however silent and guarded. Her thin, dark hair was pulled close to her head under an old-fashioned, stiff-brimmed straw hat. She wore a long, ill-fitting cotton dress. Its pattern and coarseness told that the cloth from which the garment was made had come from flour sacks. Her stockings were of a heavy brown cotton; her shoes were worn and unpolished.

I spoke a few words of greeting, held a chair for her, and then took my seat at the desk.

The hand that she rested upon the arm of her chair was thin and rough and tremulous. The nails had been bitten into the quick. Her thumb and forefinger were stained dark brown, almost black, with nicotine.

"I have been sick a long time, Doctor," she said in a low and lifeless voice. "No one knows what is the matter with me, or, if they know, they won't say what it is. One of your patients told me that you are a good doctor. I finally got my husband to bring me. Please help me."

"Let me see if I can help," I said kindly, as I resolved to do my best.

I picked up the history sheet. The first few sections had been filled in by my secretary and read as follows:

Mrs. Emma Massey
Address: RFD No. 4, City
Height: 5'3"
Weight: 98 pounds

Age: 27

Married: (<u>Yes</u>) (No)

Husband's Name: Henry L. Massey

Husband's Address: Same

Years Married: 6

No. of Children: None

Occupation: Housewife

Habits: Does not use alcohol or drugs, smokes incessantly, coffee—many cups a day

Chief Complaint: Nervousness, inability to sleep, loss of weight

Family History: Father died before she was born, killed in accident, age unknown

Mother died at age of thirty-six, when patient was a child, cause of death—pneumonia

No familial diseases that she knows of

No tuberculosis or cancer in family

Past Medical History: Except for diseases of childhood, has always been well until this trouble started

No serious illnesses or injuries

No operations

I had now come to the space under the heading, "Present Illness." This and the spaces under the printed headings which followed were blank. These were the ones I was to complete as I questioned the patient and conducted the examination.

"Tell me about your trouble," I said.

She hesitated a moment, as if trying to get her story straight, before she replied, "I began to be nervous and to feel bad about four years ago. I have got worse and worse. For the past year or two I have had headaches, and I have lost a lot of weight. I can't sleep. I have been to the doctors here, and I went down to the medical school, too, but I am getting worse all the time."

Next, I asked my patient the details of her symptoms and exactly how her illness had started. I asked if she knew any cause for the nervousness, if she had found anything that would afford relief.

She answered both questions with the one word, "No."

Upon the history sheet I wrote her statements and her answers. I mentioned various untoward symptoms and followed every lead.

Having exhausted the general questioning, I began with the various systems of the body. Starting with the head, I asked what part of the head was involved in the headache, the nature of the pain, the time of day it came, whether reading had any connection with it, and on and on. Gradually I worked down through one system after another. She answered readily enough. As I wrote each answer, I weighed its implications.

Then I asked about her home life and her happiness. She was noncommittal.

When I had finished, though I had taken a long history, I could add little significance to what she had told me at first.

Next, I very carefully examined the patient, and under the heading "Physical Examination" I recorded my almost negative findings.

By this time the reports from the laboratory examinations that I had ordered had been brought to me. They were essentially negative.

Again, we sat at my desk as I reviewed the history.

"Well," she asked anxiously, "have you found the trouble?"

I tossed the history aside.

"No, I haven't," I said as I studied her thin face with its tremulous lips.

"Do you think that there is nothing the matter with me?" she asked. "That's what my husband says."

"Yes, there is something—something bad," I replied. "At twenty-seven you should be in the prime of life, healthy and sparkling. You know the trouble. Suppose you tell me what it is. Is there something wrong at home? Is it because you want children or don't want them? What did you do before you were married? What have you done since?"

She gave a low moan. "I was hoping there was something real the matter with me," she said. "I was hoping it wasn't that."

"Tell me about it," I insisted. Perhaps I can help you, or, if you would rather, go to your minister and tell him."

After a few moments of hesitation, she told her story.

"I never had a home," she said. "All my life I wanted one. When I was a child I lived in rooming houses while my mother was off at work. After she died, I stayed on in them and worked for my keep. Then I got a place as a maid in a beauty parlor. By the time I was old enough, I had learned the work. I became an operator, made good money, and saved it. I saved it for a home.

"People said I ought not to marry Henry, that he was too old for me; but he claimed he was crazy about me and I wanted a home and children. He said that he did too, and I got to loving him. After we were married, I worked on for a while.

"Henry's sister had a little baby. Her husband had run off and left her. She had a job but didn't have any place to live. She and Henry said that if I would take my money and make the down payment on a house they would work and finish paying for it. They said that I could keep house and look after the baby and we could all live there together. They said that I could raise my own children there too.

"We bought a little place in the country where we could keep a cow and some chickens and have a garden. It was a place where I could plant some flowers and have a pretty yard.

"I always got up first because I would have to cook breakfast and pack their snacks and get them off. Then I would milk the cow and take care of the baby and the place. I kept the house nice and clean. I did the washing and ironing and everything else that was done there. When Henry and his sister came home at night they were tired, and I always cooked a good supper for them. I took care of the baby at night too, but I didn't mind that . . . then.

"When I told my husband I wanted a baby of my own, he said to wait until his sister's baby was older and we got in better shape. He wouldn't listen to anything else. I thought things would be all right after a while, so I didn't say anything more about it then.

"Well, when the baby should have begun to get up, it didn't. It grew all right and got fat, but it was two years old before it could sit up just a little. They got a doctor to see it, and he said it had a birth injury and that it would never be any better.

"My husband and his sister got so hard after that. Henry said he never wanted a baby of his own—that it might turn out like that one. I have begged him many of a time since then, but he won't listen to me.

"The little boy is six years old now. He walks about some, but he can't feed or care for himself. I have to do everything for him, night and day. He doesn't know me or anyone else. Every day he has several convulsions. Then he will take spells of beating his head against the bed or against the wall.

"I believe I could stand all that if it weren't for the cry he makes. It isn't from pain. It doesn't sound like anything else on earth. It's a long, high 'aw-aw-aw' that keeps on and on and on. It has in it all the anguish there is. Off and on all day, he makes that cry. That's bad enough, but it is the nights that are killing me. I can't stand it any longer. I can't stand to lie there in the dark with everyone else asleep and listen to that cry."

"Do you still take care of the child and do all the other work there?" I asked.

"Yes," she replied, "but I have to keep a pot of coffee on the stove and drink it all day to keep going. I don't see how I can listen to that cry anymore. Tell me what to do."

"You are young and should have a home of your own," I said. "Why don't you sell the house and divide the money? You and your husband could get a little place by yourselves."

"I tried to get them to do that. Henry won't go, and his sister says that if we leave, she will stop paying on the house and won't sell it and that I'll lose all I've put into it."

"The care of the child is its mother's responsibility, not yours," I told her. "Perhaps she can put it in some institution."

"No, she won't do that," she replied.

"Let me talk to your husband and tell him the real trouble and see if he can't work something out."

"Oh no! Don't do that. Please don't tell him that is all that is wrong with me." She looked terrified.

"Anything is better than going on like this," I said.

"No, it isn't," she replied quickly.

It crossed my mind to tell her to run away, to strike out for herself as she once had. I thought it over.

This might, I decided, have far-reaching consequences that I could not risk.

"Go to your minister and tell him about it," I suggested again.

"I have been and he can't help me."

"Then go to the judge of the police court and get him to advise you."

"I can't do that. Give me some medicine for my nerves, can't you?" she begged.

"That's just what I don't want to do," I said. "I want really to help you. While I think of it, there are two things I must tell you. One is to stop smoking so much. That makes you feel dull and depressed and gives you a headache. The other is to stop drinking so much coffee."

"The doctors at the medical school told me that cigarettes and coffee didn't cause the nervousness, that my craving them was just a symptom."

"A man in deep trouble might be distraught," I replied. "In that case an urge to shoot himself might be only a symptom but, still, it would be wiser for him to put the gun back in the drawer."

"I have to have them to keep going," she told me.

"Come back to see me a few times and let me try to build you up while I think about it," I suggested.

"No, I can't come again. Why don't you give me some medicine?"

I wrote a prescription for a mild sedative.

"What do I owe you?" she asked.

"Nothing," I told her.

"Yes, I want you to charge me. They won't think there is anything the matter with me if you don't."

I considered her request for a moment.

"Give my secretary two dollars," I replied, and she left me.

A few minutes later my secretary came to me. She was shaking with agitation as she related what had happened.

"That woman came to the desk to pay," she said. "She had a ten-dollar bill in her hand. She told me that she owed two dollars. Her husband jumped up, snatched the bill out of her hand, and without a word put it in his pocket. Then he took out two one-dollar bills and gave them to me. I wish you could have seen it."

I walked to the window and looked out. I stood and watched the backs of three figures that came from the mass of the building. One was a heavy-set, thick-necked, coarsely dressed man; one, a tall, angular woman. Between them, clutched firmly by her upper arms and being pushed and dragged along, was a thin, frail figure which reeled and staggered as they moved away, on across the paved court.

A Matter of Sequence

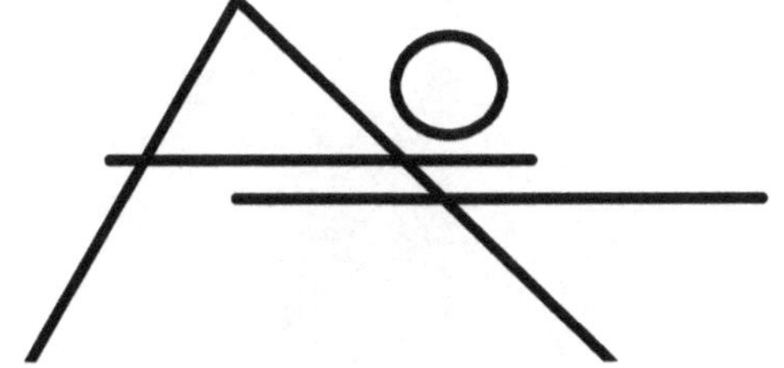

A Matter of Sequence

Lester Warren, M.D., made no bones about it. He wanted a son. The night had come for the crucial test, the last chance—or so it seemed—and I the last dependence. This was a role I did not especially fancy now that I was face to face with it.

I stood in the darkness on the platform at the ambulance entrance and waited for Dr. Warren to bring his wife to the hospital. The darkness soothed me somewhat until there in its stillness I began to put my nerves on edge afresh by recalling to mind the pertinent events of the seven years I had known them. It seemed that night as if it had been much longer—indeed, as if the world's major objective for many years had been the fulfillment of Dr. Warren's desire, and its chief sorrow his disappointments.

When I first met Dr. Warren he had, by a former wife, four daughters; had married again; and was already looking forward to what he felt would be the crowning event of his life. Soon he told me about it.

"This time it will be a boy," he said; but no, it was not. Time passed. The pregnancy proved to be abnormal.

I recommended that he take his wife to a surgeon in whom I had great confidence. He finally agreed. Later he returned to say that both he and his wife wanted me to perform the operation.

"No," I said, "we have been through all that before. You know how close I stand to you and Mrs. Warren. If something should go wrong, I would never get over it."

Nothing else would do, however, and it ended by my operating on her. She got along nicely, and it was well for my peace of mind that she did.

Another year or so passed, and he was in high hopes. It was to be a boy. Dr. Holmes, an unusually competent obstetrician, was caring for Mrs. Warren. She received all the attention it was possible to bestow upon one.

The labor was long and difficult. It seemed almost interminable to Lester and to me as we waited in the anteroom at the hospital. Hours passed. Yes, it was a boy, a beautiful, fine boy, but it was dead.

The parents—noble, wonderful people—shed no tear. There was not the slightest break in their voices. There were no words but those of gratitude to the obstetrician. They seemed bent on trying to keep him from feeling hurt. It seemed to me that I was more distressed than they.

Nothing daunted, Dr. Warren in due time informed me that they were to be given another chance.

"This time I am going to keep my wife at home and deliver her myself," he said. "I have delivered thousands of babies in their own homes. That is the safest place. I am going to have a son yet. I'll show you."

I was not invited to participate—not at first, that is. On the day of the expected delivery, I heard nothing. At midnight the telephone rang, and Lester's anxious, distressed voice asked that I pick up Dr. Holmes and come as fast as I could.

A Matter of Sequence

It was winter and the ground was covered with snow, but like mad we drove the twenty miles to the Warren home. When we arrived, I soon saw that we should not have been in such a hurry. There was a long period of waiting, just as there had been the time before.

Hour after hour passed. We walked the floor, drank coffee, and talked without knowing what was said. Dr. Holmes, who felt the direct responsibility, had been in and out of the patient's room many times. As the night wore on, he became more and more apprehensive.

"We are going to lose that baby if we wait any longer," he finally said. "I am going to proceed."

I gave the anesthetic, and Dr. Holmes delivered the baby. It was a girl this time. It never breathed.

There was now the grim and tragic air of keen disappointment, of sorrow and of bitter self-reproach on Lester's part.

"It's no use. It's no use trying again," he said. "Call the undertaker and tell him to send for it," he told someone in a harsh, dead voice.

Mrs. Warren was coming from under the anesthetic and was rational enough to hear her husband's voice, to comprehend it's meaning, but not enough to have her customary self-control. Her screams and wailing cries resounded through the house as she burst into tears. Dr. Holmes and I gathered up our instruments and started for the car. It was a cold, gray dawn.

"It's no use," Dr. Warren repeated as he walked out with us.

"Lester, there is something the matter—bad," I said. "I don't care what the x-rays and the examination show. There is some reason why she can't have a baby, or Dr. Holmes could deliver her safely. It is going to take a surgeon. Leave it to me next time. Let me do a Cesarean section on her. I'll get you a live baby."

I didn't know how deep an impression I had made on him—deep enough I found out later—for after another year he told me that he was taking me at my word and gave the approximate date when I could expect to perform the operation.

Because of Dr. Warren's anxiety, there was a period of two months or more before the day he had named when I dared not leave the telephone for more than a few minutes at a time. If for any reason he called and I was not instantly accessible, he would become almost frantic. He would call to send me a patient, he would call to tell me how his wife was doing, and he would call just to make sure that I was standing by.

He urged me to operate upon her ahead of time.

"Just to make sure," he said.

I would not do that.

At last, this night, he had called to say that his wife was in labor and that he was bringing her to the hospital at once. It chanced that I was away from the hospital at the time.

"He was quite put out," the admitting clerk told me when I came to the hospital a few minutes later. I telephoned to the Warren home, but they had already started. I told the operating room force to get everything in readiness, as there might be little time to do so after Mrs. Warren arrived.

After seeing that all arrangements were made, I had come to the ambulance platform where I now stood, waiting in the dark. Several months before, I had felt sure of myself and very sure of the outcome. As these months passed, however, this confidence slowly drained away. Now, as I stood on the platform, I felt anything but confident. I thought of the years of disappointment, of the tragic scenes that had gone before, and of the chance that this might be just another failure. Perhaps fate itself had entered the list against him and would bring every effort to naught. I became almost beside myself.

What will I do if this attempt ends like the others?" I exclaimed to myself. Well, I asked for it.

Suddenly the headlights of Dr. Warren's car flooded the area and showed him that I was waiting. Mrs. Warren was sitting beside her husband. We greeted one another warmly. To my immense relief, they did not show the slightest anxiety or fear of the outcome.

"This is the thing to do. Everything will be all right," I reassured myself.

Dr. Warren was friendly and laughing—a little too freely, perhaps. He was out of the car now and handing the luggage from the back seat. I carried Mrs. Warren's suitcase and he carried the baby basket, decked out in blue ribbons for their son. In the hospital we put these in the hall for the orderly to handle and took the elevator to the operating suite.

In the dressing room we changed our clothes, put on our white suits, and then sat down to wait until we should be notified that the patient had been brought up and that we should scrub for the operation. We spoke of other patients that Dr. Warren had in the hospital and talked about several items of civic interest. Dr. Warren told of some amusing incidents which had come to his attention since last we met. We both avoided the subject closest to our hearts. I became more and more nervous.

Finally, I said to him, "I wonder what's the matter. They should have called us long ago. I'll go and see how much longer it will be."

In the operating room everything was in order but Mrs. Warren was not there. The nurses, one dressed in her sterile gown, were standing about the room.

"Why, what's wrong?" I asked. "Why hasn't the patient been sent up?"

"We don't know," they answered.

Dr. Warren was close behind me now. We were again tense and anxious. I telephoned down to the night supervisor.

"Why hasn't Mrs. Warren been sent up?" I asked. "Dr. Warren and I are waiting."

"I didn't know that they had arrived," she said. "I'll send her up at once."

A few minutes later she telephoned. The sound of her voice indicated that she was puzzled. It also carried a trace of alarm as she said, "We can't find her anywhere. She isn't in her room."

Lester and I did not wait for the elevator. We raced down the stairs and out to the car.

There sat Mrs. Warren just as we had left her. She was laughing at us. There wasn't the slightest trace of concern. She was genuinely amused.

"I wondered how long it would be before you missed me", she said. "I don't know about the old riddle, but in these days a mother comes before a son. Now if you get me a real live boy, I'll never tell."

And she kept her promise.

The Whited Sepulcher

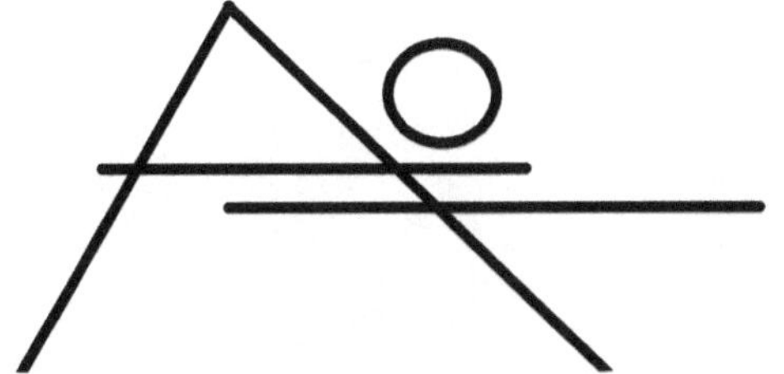

The Whited Sepulchre

It would not be an ordinary call nor would it be a pleasant one to make. I was sure of that the moment I heard those almost incoherent words over the telephone.

"This is Ruth Thomas. Come as soon as you can." There were tears in her voice and a sobbing, broken-hearted appeal.

This young woman and her husband, a very successful mining engineer, were patients of mine—a little more than that; for once I had been with them through a very trying time unrelated to medicine. I had become fond of them and had always looked upon their marriage as an example of an affectionate and loving union. It was a childless marriage, but one that I felt sure would endure. Lately, however, I had not been so certain of this. The wife had come to me with ailments that I thought were largely imaginary. She had also given me the impression that her relations with her husband were not as happy as they formerly had been. Then too, she had always been erect, spirited, and dressed in clothes of the latest fashion, appropriate for the occasion and most becoming to her. Lately she had not walked with the same lightness and had not been attired with her customary care. Her face was beginning to line, and her eyes had lost much of their luster.

So disturbed had I been during her last visit that for some time afterward I had carried in my mind a consideration as to whether or not I should ask her to come see me again in order that I might give her some helpful advice. I thought of urging her to travel with her husband on his long trips, as once she had done. Then, in the press of other duties, the matter had slipped from my mind. All this now came back to me, and I knew what to expect.

Looking for the number, I drove along the fashionable street until I came to their new house. It was set in a large lot and some distance back from the street. It was a modern, one-story, rambling structure with large picture windows, all of the most pleasing design and in palatial scale—the work of architects of the highest order.

Never have I seen a more attractive house or one in a more beautiful setting, I thought as I looked at it standing there—a misty gray in the moonlight.

I went up the steps to the door and rang the bell. The husband, Earl Thomas, came to the door. I instantly felt that, while not in any way hostile, he was somewhat sorry to see me. He took my coat and hat and led me into an interior as remarkably beautiful as the exterior of the house had seemed to me. There was only a moment to observe this, however, for now I came into the large living room, where his wife was pacing the floor.

Ruth, who had never before more than tasted whiskey, was drunk and raving. Just how much liquor there was and how much spleen would be hard to say. Without pausing, she continued her furious pace back and forth the length of the room. She was crying in rage, striking the palm of one hand with the fist of the other, and striking the furniture with such force as was likely to break the bones in her hand. At the same time, she was screaming invectives at her husband, saying that she wanted me to know what a blackguard he was and telling me of the ways he had abused her.

She was a slender and shapely woman about thirty-five years of age, slightly above the average in height, and still attractive even though the first freshness of youth had passed, even though her hair was down, which it actually as well as figuratively was. It was light brown and falling over her shoulders. Her usually mild light blue eyes were now bloodshot and flashing fire. She wore a short-sleeved housecoat which struck her just below the knees. On her feet was a pair of knitted socks with embroidered feet and soft leather soles.

Earl was a year or two older than his wife. He was a large, muscular man with strong, rather handsome features. Now his dark brown hair was tousled and his gray eyes were open very wide, staring, following the movements of his wife. His face, usually highly colored, was intensely pale. He was cold sober and in great distress. His thin lips were tightly drawn. He took a chair across from the sofa where I now sat. His wife's path lay between us.

"What in the world is the matter?" I asked.

"He didn't think I would tell you but I will," she cried, continuing with great agitation to recount her list of wrongs.

"Let me give you something so that you can sleep," I suggested. "Then settle this when you are more able to do so."

"No! I am going to tell it now. I am not going to stay in this house tonight. He threatened to kill me and would if he weren't afraid. That's why I sent for you. I want you to hear what I have to say."

"I am a friend from happier times than this," I said. "If both of you want me to stay, I will do so. If either would rather I leave, I will go now."

"Stay, Doctor. Can't you give her something?" asked the husband.

"I won't take it I tell you!" she shouted while continuing her ceaseless striding back and forth. She seized two china ashtrays from a table and hurled one to the floor as she passed going in one direction and hurled the other down as she returned. The raised figures on the edge of the ashtray thrown in the direction I chanced to be looking shattered as it struck the floor while the heavy bowl, unbroken, bounced into a radio set, scarring it slightly.

The husband arose and with a sponge and bottle of cleaning fluid, which he produced from nowhere as he left his chair, scrubbed a spot from the otherwise immaculate rug, gathered up the broken pieces of the ashtrays, and ruefully eyed the scar on the cabinet.

"That radio cost a thousand dollars," he said.

"That's just it! He thinks more of the house and the furniture than he does of me!" shouted the wife. "It's all for show, not to live in. I can't sit down in here for fear I will mess up the room. I have to go into the den. My little dog can't come into the house for fear he will get a hair on a cushion."

She struck the sofa I was sitting on with her fist and something on her hand left a wet spot. Instantly, the husband sprang up with his sponge and cleaning fluid.

The woman strode by, throwing her feet out stiff-legged in her fury. Her socks kept coming halfway off and she kept pulling them on again.

"I pressed his clothes and turned his shirt collars and cuffs when he had nothing," she said. "Now that he is successful and making money, he won't give any of it to me. He has had three new cars in the last six months, and when I say something about it, he tells me that he makes the money and will spend it as he pleases. He hates me because I have a little money of my own and won't give it to him."

The husband injected, "One of those cars was defective, and another was torn up in a wreck. I have to have a good car. I drive all the time."

"Yes, he drives all the time," she shouted, "and I stay at home waiting for him, and when he comes, he sits around and drinks and sleeps. He never feels like talking to me or playing golf with me or taking me anywhere. I used to travel with him but I gave it up. I gave it up the day he told me that he felt ashamed of my appearance when I came to the table at a hotel where some of his friends were dining. I can't travel in a car for days and have a freshly pressed dress every time we stop.

"That's the way I have been treated, and now he blames it all on sex," she cried. "He says we are not getting along because we are unsuited in that way. That has to come naturally with me. I can't be forced. When I told him so, he said he was going out and get a hussy. I slapped him, which he deserved, and he threatened to kill me."

"Speak up," she said to her husband. "Tell him if it isn't true."

"No, no, that won't do," I said, shaking my head. "That's the stuff tragedy is made of. As for the other, I know it is said that such an adjustment is of paramount importance in a happy marriage; but from what I have seen I believe that of much greater importance are unselfishness, understanding, and the underlying devotion of a man and his wife to each other. If each is trying to make the other happy, these other relations will take care of themselves."

Of course, I had not been entirely dumb even before I ventured this last observation, but had from time to time put in such comments and offered such advice as I thought might make for a reconciliation.

"You were both much happier," I now said, "when you were turning cuffs and each thinking of the other instead of your possessions.

How long have you had this place? May I see the other rooms?" I asked to divert them somewhat.

The husband took me on a tour. The entire interior was most attractive. In some of the rooms one or more of the walls were painted, and the other walls of these same rooms were done in the finest scenic wallpaper. The kitchen was of the most modern design, colorful and pretty. I was shown the various gadgets and new features. Each of the bedrooms had a dressing room and a bath, all shining in plate glass and chrome, with matched sets of luxurious accessories. In one dressing room were closets with rows and rows of pretty dresses and dozens of pairs of pretty shoes.

"She has an account at every store in town and a new car of her own," the husband said.

In the closets of his room were guns, golf clubs, riding boots, and all those things a well-to-do man accumulates.

I passed a nice bar, well stocked—too well, I thought.

By the time the tour was complete, the wife had quieted down. Enough time had passed for her to sober somewhat.

Then, too, she was interested in the attention I was giving the house.

"I found the material for the living room curtains myself," she spoke up when I admired them.

"This is a beautiful house," I said, returning to my place on the sofa, "and very handsomely furnished, but it looks as if everything still wears its price tag. I liked the old home better. This one will have to have a lot of living in and many a stain and worn place and scratch and scar before it looks as good as the other. You can, with money, build a beautiful house and furnish it; but it takes caring for one another, unselfishness, and love to make a home. Can't you see that it lies within both of you to make this place a hell, as it is tonight, or to make it a sanctuary, a haven—a heaven?"

Neither of them spoke nor moved now. In my own earnestness and emotion, I did not look at them.

"A home is here for the taking if both of you see its importance, desire it, and work for it," I continued, "but it cannot be if one selfishly tries to impose his or her will on the other. This kind of scene doesn't happen all at once. It is the final bursting out of pent-up emotions repressed a long time.

"Can't you see that all this prosperity has no substance, that the intangible bond between you is the only thing that counts—the knowledge that your wife is waiting for you when you start home, Earl, and then that your husband is coming home to you, Ruth; the light in your eyes when you look at each other; the thrill of touching hands; the knowledge that there is in the world, after all, one person who is yours and all for you? That is how it was when I first knew you. You have missed the real thing somewhere along the way."

Without any leave-taking that I remember, I asked for my hat and coat. I was thoroughly exhausted. After climbing into my car, I looked back at the house. I was reminded of those "whited sepulchers, which indeed appear beautiful outward, but are within full of dead men's bones."[3]

I heard nothing more from the Thomases. Several weeks passed before I was in that neighborhood again. I went a little out of my way in order to go by their house. As I drove along, I debated as to whether or not I should stop. I did, but not to visit them. A large "For Sale" sign was nailed to a tree near the street. The curtains were drawn. There was no sign of life.

---

3. Acts 23:3 (King James Version).

The Scar

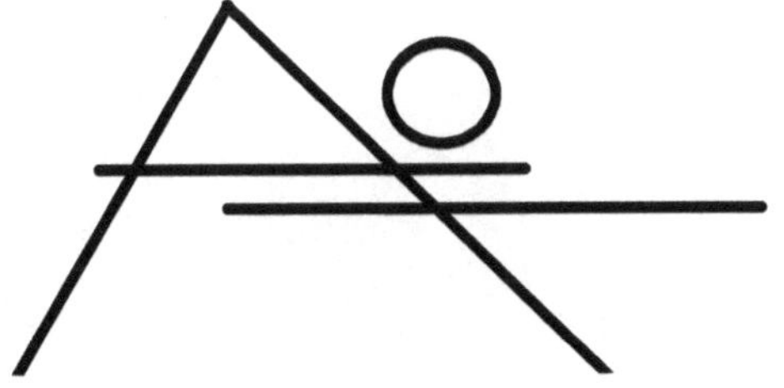

The Scar

Near a village built around a large mill a narrow, grassy strip wound upward between two hills.

Up this vale a great power line passed on its way to the mill. Ranging up the slopes on each side was a number of small houses. On the green the children played, and in certain areas the day's wash fluttered from the numerous wire lines that were used in common by several families. There was little to foretell the drama that was to be enacted there that spring morning.

Walking about in search of a suitable location for a radio aerial, Tom Van Horn looked this way and that and finally decided that from his house he could stretch the wire high over the power line to a tree on the opposite slope. Relying on the insulation for safety, he tied a stone to one end of his wire and, holding the other end in his left hand, threw the stone over the power line. The great wires instantly burned the insulation, burned themselves in two, fell upon and charged a tangle of clotheslines. Van Horn received the full charge and terribly burned, fell in agony, crying for help.

From a house across the green, a man named Deering ran to his assistance. Deering's chest struck a clothesline. Like some giant cleaver, the line sliced through his ribs and lung. As he fell, he struck another line that sliced off the upper part of his head. He still lived and thrashed about in agony.

Deering's wife, so I was told, ran up. She seemed to know that she should not touch the wires or the charged bodies beneath them. Dashing frantically here and there, waving a sweater high above her head, she threw one end of the sweater over a line and instantly paid for this indiscretion with her life. She fell dead, her clothes ablaze.

In the few minutes while this scene was being enacted, someone telephoned Dr. Howard Craig at his office in the village. He sprang into his car and raced to the scene of the accident. Dr. Craig took in the situation at a glance—the long, black streaks in the green grass; the stench of burning flesh; the writhing, groaning men; the smoldering form of the woman—all upon and beneath the tangled, deadly wires.

Dr. Craig was a strong and resourceful man, intelligent and careful. At the same time, he was fearless and selfless. Seizing a rake which was standing nearby, he crawled on his hands and knees under the crackling, snapping, swaying wires which were still falling in places. Avoiding those hanging ends, the deadly clothes whipping in the breeze and the wires on the ground, he used the rake to roll the victims off the charged lines. He took hold of the most badly injured man, Deering, and dragged him from that tragic stage. One ambulance had arrived and Dr. Craig loaded Deering into it and sent it on its way. Then, without a second's hesitation, he turned and crawled back under the wires for the others.

An excited voice over the telephone told us that the first ambulance was making the twenty-mile run to the hospital. Preparations in the operating room had hardly been completed before the ambulance swung into the drive and up to the emergency door. The patient, moaning and thrashing about in his dying agony, was whisked into the elevator and up to the operating room. Never had I seen a more terrible sight. He expired within a few minutes.

The ambulance driver had come up with the patient, had stood by, and now described the accident. It is his version that I have given. The driver further stated that I could expect the second ambulance at any minute and indeed, at that instant, we heard the scream of its siren.

Dr. Craig and I followed the stretcher into the operating room. Van Horn seemed more dead than alive. He was in shock. His left arm was burned to a crisp well above the elbow and there was a great charred area over one shoulder blade, another upon the sole of one foot. We amputated the arm above the line of the burn, cut out the charred areas, and treated him for shock.

After finishing, Dr. Craig and I went into the dressing room. As we changed our clothes, we talked of the accident.

"The ambulance driver told me that Deering's wife was killed," I said.

"No, it was Van Horn's wife who was killed," said Dr. Craig. "You remember Mrs. Van Horn. You operated on her for a goiter. She got entirely well. She had a beautiful scar. I looked at it today."

"Ah!" I said, deeply moved. "Isn't that too bad! Of course, I remember her."

Mrs. Van Horn had been one of the first patients who came to me after I started practice in the city. Because of this and because she had been so ill, I remembered her well. Now my mind, in its over-wrought state, pictured her in all the sharpness and clarity of life.

She had been a tall, large-boned woman and had always dressed in plain and somber clothes. Her enormous brown eyes, because of the disease, almost protruded from their sockets. With them, as I talked to her, she was wont to fix me with a most disquieting stare. The skin of her face was sallow and hung in folds. Her salt-and-pepper hair was exceedingly coarse.

The operation on her goiter had been difficult and dangerous. It had to be done in two stages and I had not been especially proud of the scar.

"He knows it was the best that could have been done under the circumstances," I said to myself.

She is gone, I thought, as my mind pictured every detail of her features.

In silence, Dr. Craig and I finished dressing and, taking the elevator, dropped to the floor where Mr. Van Horn had been taken.

Dr. Craig sat down at the nurses' desk and began to look through the charts of other patients he had in the hospital. He seemed calm enough, but I was shaken and unnerved.

"I'll be back in a minute. I want to see how he is doing," I said.

I walked to the patient's room, gave a slight tap, and opened the door. Several persons were standing between the bed and me.

"Here's the doctor," someone said in a low tone, and the visitors began to step aside to allow access to the injured man.

One glance showed Mr. Van Horn propped up in bed, comfortable and out of danger. A further movement allowed my eyes to move to a form standing beyond and close to him. It was

The Scar

Mrs. Van Horn, as plain as I had just seen her in my mind, as plain as she had ever stood in life. Of all those in the room, she alone neither moved nor spoke. She stood at the head of the bed and stared at me with her great protruding eyes. I stopped in my tracks. I felt the surge of my heart, a constriction in my chest, a numbness. My eyes, widening, took in every detail of her form—the strong, coarse hair; the sagging, sallow face—all lifelike, refreshing my memory and correcting slightly the mental picture I had just reviewed. There was the scar! None of the others seemed to have seen her; they were turning to me. Dr. Craig was not a man to make a mistake. He said she was dead yet there she stood.

The very floor seemed an unsubstantial thing under my feet. Those around me dropped out of focus like wraiths and I looked into a spectral world without boundary between substance and shadow.

Half-crouched, every faculty was straining to its highest pitch. With eyes burning, piercing, I attempted in vain to penetrate through and beyond that vacant stare. Step by step, I backed out of the room and closed the door.

Swiftly I strode up the hall. By the time I reached the desk, my mind was settling on the obvious explanation.

"It was Mrs. Deering, not Mrs. Van Horn—I mean the one that was killed," I said.

"No, it was Mrs. Van Horn," said Dr. Craig. "You remember Mrs. Van Horn, don't you? You operated upon her for a goiter. I looked at her scar today."

"I tell you Mrs. Van Horn is in that room," I almost shouted, pointing down the hall.

His eyes searched my own. With a sudden movement he came to his feet. Together we hurried to the door. Dr. Craig opened it, took one glance, and closed it.

"That's Mrs. Van Horn all right," he said, but it's not the one. That's his brother's wife. You operated on both of them for goiter."

The Last Will and Testament

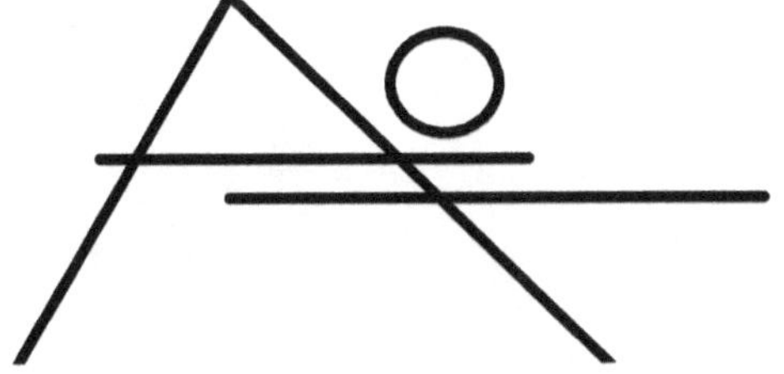

The Last Will and Testament

"Come on! Out with it! You can soft-soap some folks, but I want the truth. You have the letter from that fancy doctor you sent me to. Am I going to get well or not?"

As I looked into my patient's cold, steely-gray eyes, I realized that she meant what she said—that I could not evade the issue. I slowly shook my head.

"You knew it all the time, didn't you?" she demanded.

"Yes," I replied.

Her countenance did not change.

Until lately she had been a handsome woman of beautiful physique and with a certain delusive charm. Recently her glamour had faded considerably—not that Edna Grey had ceased to be a woman of striking appearance. Let no one be mistaken about that.

A master might have cut her long, perfectly straight nose and her clear features from a block of Carrara marble, I thought; and as I did so, it occurred to me that she was, indeed, about that cold.

Now she spoke again. Her voice was clear and decisive as she said, "Come to see me tomorrow afternoon. I want to talk to you—at four o'clock if that suits you."

The chauffeur held the door as I handed her into the limousine. He closed the door, took his seat, and awaited her signal; but Edna Grey did not sink back into the luxurious interior. She leaned toward the open window. Her black velvet collar, secured at the throat by a large diamond brooch, flared upward. Above it her face seemed intensely white. She cared more than she would have me believe.

"Just when you have everything fixed and think you are ready to live," she said, "you have to lay it all down."

With the speed of light, the happenings of years went through my mind. Involuntarily, I took a step or two backward. As I looked away from her, the shiny hubcap of the car caught my eye and, in some strange fascination, I watched it turn slowly, over and over, and pass out of the line of my vision. A moment later the spell passed, and I turned toward my office.

I had known the first Mrs. Grey, the real one. She was tall and willowy and lovely. She had come straight from a finishing school to be Weston Grey's bride.

"What a wonderful choice he has made!" all of his friends said, and they were right.

She too had light eyes, but they were a soft, kindly blue with a touch of violet in them. She had all the quiet composure, the bearing, and the stateliness of a queen.

Weston had been considered the most eligible bachelor in our town. He was finely educated, gentle, and trained to social perfection. Also, being the sole heir, he had come early into the ownership of the Grey ancestral home and the family's wealth.

"Fine looking too," all said at first.

Later, when the charm of boyhood had passed, he should have developed into a handsome man but did not. With this, we had reason for thought and to make comparisons, and he began to appear in a somewhat different light. We then began to notice his small, upturned nose, faded eyes, and thin, dimpled chin. He wore a small mustache, pointed and waxed at the tips. I never saw him without his slender cane. No, Weston was not the equal of his fathers. Biologically, he was a sport, just as Edna was a sport compared with the other members of her family.

"Strong or weak," one of his closest friends said to me, "I can never understand how he could become entangled with his peroxide-blonde secretary and endanger his relations with his own beautiful wife and two lovely children."

Weston did just this, however.

A divorce was arranged. Mrs. Grey obtained full possession of the little boy and girl. For this she surrendered much in a material way. Weston made a hard and parsimonious bargain with her. I was told that Edna, with her indomitable will, was the force behind his maneuvers.

Mrs. Grey and her two children moved away. Weston married Edna. None of the Greys' former friends ever called. Weston and his new wife kept to themselves. One by one, he dropped his memberships in his clubs and gave up his old activities.

One May I walked with him along a path on his estate. He swung his slender, gold-headed cane and decapitated every flower he chanced upon. He had developed an incurable and progressive illness. I had purposely led him from the house to tell him I had learned that through an unfortunate turn in the market of the depression years his former wife and his children were in very poor financial circumstances. Weston said he would talk with Edna and see what could be done. Nothing was done. He seemed to have no power to think or act for himself.

In all cases which are to have a fatal termination, the day, put off for a while or not, soon comes around. Weston's days were checked off one by one until all were gone. He left his home, his personal and real property, and every dollar he possessed to Edna. There was no entailment. Those vast properties that his forefathers had built simply passed from his family. He had sold not only his own birthright, but also that of his children for a mess of pottage.

And now it was Edna's turn—her turn to button her coat all the way to the chin and ready herself to step forward when her name was called.

The next afternoon, at the gatehouse of the Grey Estate, as the old keeper greeted me, I noticed a quietness as compared with his cheerfulness of former times. He swung back the great iron gates, each with its tracery of foliage and of a buck rearing full length, turning and extending his graceful, antlered head upward as he sought to reach an iron cluster of wild grapes. The gates portrayed the very spirit of the park and told of the elegance that lay beyond.

The drive wound through the autumn woods, past oaks with their splotchy red and green leaves, past golden hickories, brilliantly colored berries and shrubs, and dark, shadowy hemlocks. Somewhere along the way a Great Dane had joined me, silently loping beside the car. Rounding a curve, I came in sight of the house amid its clump of giant oaks.

It was a large brick structure, now well covered with ivy. It might have been considered Early Georgian, though its large fenestrations and many double-glass doors opening upon terraces gave to it much more grace and lightness than is usually associated with that style of architecture. English boxwoods, yews and azaleas flanked the house, marked out the walks and followed the walls of the garden.

I stopped and alighted from my car. The great dog stood to one side, as motionless as a statue, and watched me climb the steps.

The old butler—white-haired and bent—opened the door. He had known me in the days when I was a frequent visitor there and his rather tired face lit up. A moment later his wife came from the rear hall to speak to me and shake my hand.

I glanced about the great paneled hall at the portraits of members of the once-proud family. The house seemed to be furnished just as I had seen it last, with the finest examples of period furniture, antique rugs, and rare accessories, yet it seemed strangely empty. The material forms were there, but life and soul were not. I was shown into the library, with its banks of thousands of volumes of books bound in rich-colored leather, embossed and lettered in gold.

Standing before the blazing log fire, I looked up at the portrait above the mantel.

Yes, this is the one Weston's little boy resembles, I thought. He resembles this man who founded the empire. Now, that little boy, the flesh and blood of this man in the portrait—his namesake—is homeless and without any means with which to secure an education, perhaps in actual want.

Edna came in. Without a word of greeting she began, "You turned away as I tried to talk to you yesterday." She was not angry but she was very serious.

"Did I do that?" I parried.

"You know you did," she replied, "and I know very well why. All last night I lay awake and thought about it. I wanted you to come so that I might ask how long you think I can live and to get you to tell me what I might expect, but that can wait. Now I am more interested in talking about the things that went through my mind last night. First it was Weston, and now it is I. It is as if some unseen hand has been laid on us. Where did my plans go wrong?"

"Are you sure your plans were not wrong to start with?" I ventured.

Her cold, gray eyes, without wavering, gazed into my own. "I learned life the hard way," she said. "I succeeded when I finally made up my mind to stop at nothing in advancing my own fortune—to do what everyone does, the best thing for oneself—regardless of any and all others. All who have wealth have been ruthless. It is remembered against an individual or even a family for a while and then it is forgotten."

I did not answer and her eyes turned downward, not in remorse but in thought. She looked toward the window and out over the grounds.

How could those cold, hard eyes and that superficial beauty have attracted Weston? I wondered. As I looked, her face began to lighten, a note of merriment such as I had not seen there before came to her perfect features. Her eyes began to kindle, a twinkle came to their corners, and a smile burst forth, animated and radiant.

"I can prove that I haven't been very bad," she said. "You believe, don't you Doctor, that only the good die young?"

This animation had come from her attempt at a poor joke! Yes, those eyes could lighten. In her desire and passion, they could and had become fire and tow to destroy. They had destroyed Weston and before that, I had been told, stronger men than he.

"No, they are the ones who live," I said. "The ones who die young are those who dissipate their lives—those who break the laws of health, of nature, of man, and of God."

She was white now, tense, and very serious. "I can understand only some of that," she said.

"Neither can I understand all of it," I replied, "but still I believe it—that life or death is there in the seed we sow."

She gripped the arms of her chair and leaned forward.

"How can that be?" she asked. She waited as I turned it over in my mind.

"You believe that an act of wisdom from its very nature leads to its own reward, don't you?" I asked at last.

"Yes," she replied.

"I believe," I said, "that not only such acts; but also every action has within it its own inherent retribution, whether it be reward or punishment. Evil carries the seed of its own destruction. So quietly, so naturally do these grow that those who eat their bitter fruit are often unaware of its source. Likewise, the blessings one reaps are not often recognized as the product of the nobility from which they sprang."

She weighed every word. When I had finished, she turned her gaze to the fire. After a few minutes she gave a slight moan. It seemed partly from pain, partly from the weariness of the soul that had stolen upon her in that night of wakefulness.

"Doctor, please come tomorrow. I want you to keep me from suffering."

"Then why not . . ." I began.

"No, tomorrow," she broke in.

"I will send you a prescription," I insisted. "The directions will be on the bottle."

She let it go at that, and I left her.

The next day I was shown upstairs. Clad in a housecoat, Edna sat before the fire. She had visitors I had not seen before. One was her old mother. In her brow and manner was a faint resemblance to Edna. She was somewhat stooped. Her worn brown dress was long out of style. She pulled off a frayed woolen glove to shake hands with me. She too had light eyes, but they were a soft, kindly blue with a touch of violet in them. In her eyes was an expression that told of her deep anxiety for her daughter. Several times she started to bring up the subject but didn't quite dare. The others present were Edna's sister and her three children. One of these was a very pretty little girl.

"She is named for Edna," the child's mother said proudly. From the tone of her voice, I felt that she was also expressing a hope for the future.

Tea was being served. There was the antique repousse tea service which I had admired so much in the years that had passed. Edna handed me a Coalport cup. It was decorated with medallions of flowers painted in bright colors and gold upon a background of apple green, a cup worthy of any museum on earth.

The company soon left. With some insistence and prompting from the nurse, Edna now told me of her new symptoms.

Every day I visited her. The visits were sometimes short, sometimes long. Most of them were unnecessary but she insisted upon them all. Edna's favorite seat was an armchair by the window. Here I often found her looking wistfully upon the garden or out upon a vista of the distant mountains to the varying shades of the purple and violet ranges, which overlapped one another to form a frame and foil for the pale blue line of a distant lake.

As time passed, Edna became more and more depressed. Sometimes, though seated at the window, she would only sit and stare without seeing, as if deep in thought. The day came when she did not want to be lifted from the bed. I suggested that she go to the hospital, but she would not consent to this.

Now Edna's people began to come in earnest—uncles and aunts and cousins and friends. After a while she saw very few of them, but they sent up their names and notes of affection together with the flowers or other offerings they had brought.

The house and its furnishings greatly interested these newcomers. I could see them pulling down the books and putting them back and handling the articles on the desks and mantels. One day while I waited in the library, Edna's brother-in-law sat across the table from me. With his finger he poked and turned a Barye bronze of a hound killing a hare.

"I wonder what Mr. Grey wanted with that?" he said.

None of Edna's kin were near her equal either in looks or intelligence. As I have said, by some strange combination of inheritance she had varied widely from her family type.

Many of Edna's visitors came frequently, attempting to recall themselves to her mind and to her favor.

There are lots of them, I thought, but enough wealth is in this fortune their kinswoman has picked up to make each and every one rich—by their standards.

When this thought crossed my mind, it occurred to me that there was also enough for Weston's children. Enough to help them would never be missed. Having bided my time and waited for a propitious moment, I cautiously broached the subject to Edna. She shook her head with such finality that I quickly let the matter drop.

As Edna became worse, her people, out of declared concern for her, began to sit up in the house through the night. Now there were rooms full of smoke. There were whisky bottles on the tables and men with coats and shoes off sitting in easy chairs or asleep on the couches.

Edna's depression deepened. Thin and weak, she sat propped up in bed. It was not the view that interested her now. It was her wan hands, which she held up and turned before her eyes.

"Why does it have to be?" she repeated over and over again. Now more than once she asked of me, "Do you really think there is anything in what you said?"

One day when I went to see her, the butler requested that I wait a few minutes before going up. Presently, Mr. Grey's old friend and attorney came down the stairs. Later I learned that he had been called in to write Edna's will.

The deathwatch of Edna's relatives continued. One morning before daybreak, as I passed through the hall, a voice called to me from the drawing room. Glancing through the door, I saw a man in his shirtsleeves. He was sitting at a table peeling an apple. His left hand dropped the fruit and its peel upon the table as his right hand flipped the knife over so that it rested on the point with the sharp edge rotated outward. The man's thumb and forefinger slid downward upon the blade.

The Last Will and Testament

With a swinging motion he brought his forearm upward, cocked his wrist; and with a swift movement such as that used in throwing a dart, drove the point of the long, thin blade into the polished top of the mahogany table. The entire series of movements, as deft as if performed by a sleight of-hand artist, took but a single second of time. The knife stood quivering. Its owner pushed back his chair, arose, and wiped his palms on his shirt as he came toward me. Gawkily, he held out his hand.

"Edna is worse tonight, Doctor," he said. "Do all you can for her. We'll see that you get your money."

Yes, she was worse, indeed, much worse. Again, I urged her to go to the hospital where she could receive better care. Again, she refused.

Soon now she could not take fluids and would not allow me to give them by vein.

"What is the use?" she asked and then said to me, "I don't want you to do anything to prolong my life one hour. I have suffered enough."

Without fluid the end came quickly. Later I was told me of the strange and moving scene enacted the day the will was read.

Edna's relatives were now eager to learn what part of that vast estate each would receive. The day the will was read they came from far and near. The large room was full of them, smoking and whispering to one another and stretching their necks to hear.

The old attorney read the will. It's one, brief provision fell upon them like a thunderclap.

"I hereby give and bequeath all of my property, both real and personal, in equal share to Nancy Grey, first wife of my late husband, and to her two children, Charles and Elizabeth."

The Gift

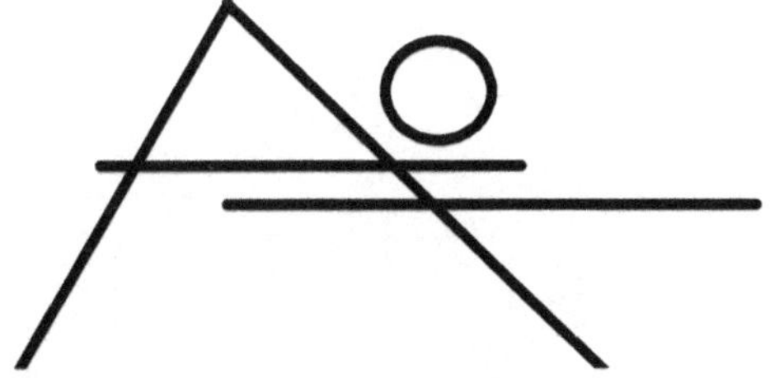

The Gift

It was Christmas Eve. With the avowed purpose of giving pleasure to one of my little patients; but perhaps more truly with the hope of regaining for a brief time some happiness from the past, of fanning the embers of a memory into life again, I hastened down the street.

It was as if a ceiling of black cloth had been stretched at the level of the reflectors over the arc lights so impenetrable was the sky above; but below these reflectors the arcs, together with the gaudy signs, lighted shops, and flaming torches of the peddlers' carts, made bright the teeming street. A misty rain fell through the light and from the mirrored surface of the pavement cast the color back again.

Shrill whistles and the ringing of bells mingled with and heightened the din of the constant honking and clatter of cars, the jazz songs, and the harsh noise of the radios. The blast of a toy trumpet sounded in my ear and its hawker cried the price and held the horn out to me as I struggled away from him through the crowd. A man stumbled and fell against me. Innumerable revelers ate from paper bags, burst them with loud reports, and threw them underfoot.

Past smoky pool rooms where youths bent over green tables or loitered in the doorway; past a throng that had collected to watch a fight; past foul-smelling fish stalls and markets where shabbily dressed men and women with cautious eyes and eager hands bought tomorrow's food; past weariness, anxiety, and haste, I strove until I reached the tenement and climbed the stairs . . . up—up until I came to my patient's room.

As I entered, the infant ceased to beat upon the floor with his spoon. Lusterless were his eyes and soiled were his pasty face, hands, and dress. After a few moments he gained his feet and tottered to the package that I had untied and pushed toward him. Into his own hands he took it and pulled from it the tinsel string. The present, which I had selected with so much care, was thrown aside. It was the crimson wrapper that had caught his fancy. Crawling backwards, he dragged it across the floor and under a table. There he sat, regarding it intently, shaking it, chewing its corner, listening to its crackling sound as he rumpled and crushed it between his hands. Never a glance did he have for the offering around which it was wrapped.

From the street the noise of the revel continued. I could distinguish every sound and picture its source.

The old Christmas feeling that I had hoped for was not revived, but as I listened to the celebration, a new thought came. Busy with it I walked to the window. Above was the abyss of the sky with its wonders and its mysteries from which came the gift of Christmas. Below the reflectors lay the world in which we live—babies, all of us, playing with the crimson paper and the silver string.

The Mask

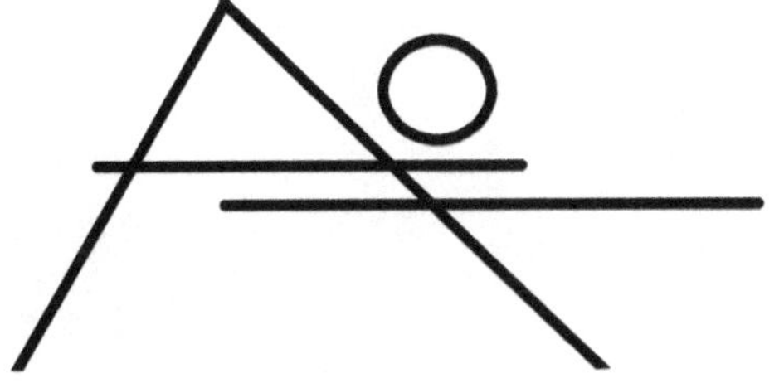

The Mask

"Who is she?" asked my secretary as she came into my private office to hand me a visiting card. "Never have I seen anyone like this woman. She says it is a social visit, that she is an old friend of yours, and if you can see her, she will wait."

I glanced at the card. Upon it was a name I did not know. Below this, written in pencil, was the simple name Eva Bentley.

"I want to see her very much," I said. "Don't let her leave. Why do you think she is so unusual?"

"I don't know what it is—some strange expression in her face," my secretary replied as she groped for an explanation. "The patients in the waiting room can't take their eyes from her."

After finishing the task at hand, I sat down at my desk and picked up her card. Swiftly, her long story passed through my mind.

It had been more than thirty years since that day when Eva had left high school to marry Herbert Bentley. She was at that time a slender, pretty girl, several inches above the average height. Her features were even and pleasant. Trusting friendliness and childlike simplicity lay in her large, soft-brown eyes. Brown hair fell in a waving mass to her shoulders. Her smooth white skin, devoid of any rosiness, was the type so harmonious with such coloring. No one could tell from a glance at her graceful, beautiful hands with their long, smooth, tapering fingers how competent they were or of how many years of service they were to perform. Her voice was quiet and distinct—each word rounded out before she was through with it. The way she dressed reflected some of those slight oddities often seen in the dress of high school girls.

Her husband, just twice her age at that time, was what might be called a man-about-town—a man about many towns, in fact; for in his work as an advance agent for a carnival he traveled far and wide.

Not long after the wedding, gossip—and even letters—describing his social activities began to drift to Eva from various sources. One of these letters was from a woman who stated that she was the mother of a child, a little girl, by Eva's husband and demanded that he take the child or provide for its support.

Confronted with the letter, Herbert acknowledged the truth of the statement. He told his wife that all this had taken place before he met her and promised that this phase of his life was now over. She in her turn said that she loved her husband enough to love his child and asked that the little girl be adopted and brought into their home. This request was at first met with indifference on her husband's part. When it was brought up again and again and insisted upon, it was finally met with a violent outburst of anger.

The matter was dropped.

As time moved on, Eva found that Herbert was not a steady worker, that he was an inconstant, one might almost say capricious, provider. Three years passed in a desultory and uncertain fashion and then came the great event of Eva's life. It was the birth of her own son, whom she named for his father.

The father did not display the same delight as did the mother. He did, however, honor his son's birth in a material way by entering into a contract, which, though it seemed to Eva somewhat out of character for him, delighted her no end. This contribution was an endowment insurance policy on his son's life. It was for a large amount, enough to give Herbert Junior a college education and a good start in any profession he might choose. It was made payable to the child in two installments, one upon his eighteenth and the other upon his twenty-first birthday. Herbert, excluding his wife as usual, had himself named as beneficiary in case of the death of his son. Through all the changing fortunes of the following years, Herbert paid the premiums and kept this policy in force.

Even though the material support Eva received from her husband became more and more meager and he, on his infrequent trips home, showed less and less concern for his wife and son, Eva's love for the child made these next few years happy ones; for, as she once said to me, the richness of life lies in giving love rather than in receiving it.

Blow after blow struck by indifference, affairs with other women, and downright brutality drove the wedge that separated the man and wife. As these two were carried farther and farther apart, Eva turned more to the boy and bestowed upon him not only a mother's love, but also all that ardor and devotion that normally would have belonged to her husband, and because of his actions were denied their natural outlet.

In order to obtain for herself and her child some sense of security, she knew that she must seek employment. Just how she could work away from home and at the same time be with her little son presented no problem to this resourceful woman. She made her decision, put in her application, and soon obtained work in the day nursery run by the city welfare department. Mother and son went together each day.

The officials of the department told me that Eva was an ideal person for this work. She was neat, orderly, of a buoyant disposition, and gave to the little children attention far beyond the call of duty. She had the knack of buying the most nutritious food for little money and, being a good cook, prepared this food well and served it in a most appetizing manner. Seeing the need, she set herself the task of learning to sew. Many a needy child received a dress or coat from Eva. Far into the night she would work, altering garments from old ones donated by a charitable organization.

The little boy grew and developed, as did his mother's love for him. Mother and son were inseparable. She adored him.

One July he became six years old. His entry into public school that fall would bring their life together at the nursery to an end. Again, she planned ahead, and by the time her son started school she had completed her arrangements. The living quarters she found had a large yard and were on a quiet side street where the little boy could safely be picked up at the door by the school bus. The rooms were in the home of an elderly widow whom Eva engaged to care for the child after school until she could be free.

This new arrangement proved most satisfactory. There were a number of children in the neighborhood and little Herbert, loving people as his mother did, made friends among them. When Eva was not at the nursery, she was with her son and his playmates. She taught them to spin tops and to fly kites. She showed them how to make valentines. She romped with them and entered into their games. In the evening she helped her son with his schoolwork.

The father's visits home became more and more rare and finally ceased. By mutual consent he and Eva separated. He went to the Far West and established his residence there.

After the two years of required separation had passed, Eva applied for a divorce. When the necessary papers were sent to Herbert, he wrote her attorney that he would not contest the divorce if a provision were made that should he ever return to the state he would have a right to demand that young Herbert spend part of his summer vacation with him. Eva told me later that she would not have consented to this had she had the slightest idea that Herbert would ever return. Her attorney treated this important detail as one of little consequence. Agreement on this point was the easy, quick way of avoiding an unpleasant ordeal in court. The failure to fight this, to take every precaution, proved to be the deciding factor that changed the course of her life.

Eva was not well when the divorce was, at length, made final. It was shortly afterwards, in the April before her son's tenth birthday in July, that she again came to me professionally. Without any feeling of self-pity, she had already written off the failure of her marriage with the deep conviction that, though things might conceivably have been better, fate had blessed her in an inordinate way—it had fulfilled her fondest dream in giving her a son. Now she was dreaming again. Her son was doing unusually well in school and she was looking forward to the time when she could go with him to the university.

It had been some time since I had seen Eva. Though she had kept her girlish spontaneity, friendliness, and much of her youthful carriage and figure, the growth and maturity of her character were plainly evident. I soon saw, however, that the most remarkable thing about her was the depth of her devotion to her child. This pervaded and shone through all else. When I told her that she must have a serious operation, her first thoughts were for the care of her son while she should be away.

Knowing her story and seeing now again the handsome little boy gave me a more than usual interest in the mother and son. One evening while Eva was in the hospital, I went for the boy and carried him to see his mother. After she had returned home and was convalescing, I again went to visit them.

A few weeks later, while I was walking along the street, a pair of patent leather half boots with white leather stitching at the top and tassels hanging down in front attracted my attention. I smiled as I saw that Eva was the one wearing them. She stopped to talk to me; she was worried. Herbert had returned from the West and had immediately demanded the custody of his son.

Herbert didn't want him for himself," she said. "He just wanted to take him away from me. He took him to his father's place in the mountains, forty miles away, and then came straight back to town. Herbert has him until the fifteenth of July and then I have him for the rest of the year. The fourteenth is his birthday. He will be ten years old. I wanted so much to have a party for him. At first Herbert said no, but when I begged, he finally said that he would bring him back for it. He hemmed and hawed so much about it though, and acted so queerly, that I am afraid he won't."

In some way I felt sorely troubled by what she had said, and my mind was filled with uneasiness long after we had separated.

Will she never be through with Herbert Bentley? Will she ever be at peace? I asked myself.

It was late afternoon of the day of the birthday party when I was next called to see her. The yard and porch were full of frightened, screaming, crying children. A birthday cake with candles all awry was on the table of the deserted living room. My eyes swept the room and took in its confusion. Chairs were overturned and presents, wrapped with colored paper and tied with ribbons, were strewn upon the floor.

Hearing the sound of a voice, I called Eva's name and went to the open door of her room. She laid face downward across the bed. The old woman with whom she lived was bending over her.

"He is dead," Eva slowly said when I spoke to her.

"Who?" I asked.

"O God in Heaven!" was all that she could say.

"What has happened? Who is dead?" I asked again.

"Her boy," answered the old woman. "Herbert was just here. He left her boy's body at the undertaking parlor. Herbert's clothes were soddened with his son's blood. It was all over his hands."

Little by little the story came out. Herbert and his brother-in-law, with whom he stayed, had borrowed guns and driven to Herbert's old home in the mountains. Having told the boy that they were going hunting and having asked him to go along, they took him into the deep woods, far from the house. At length Herbert and his son sat down upon a log to rest. The brother-in-law circled around the knoll where they sat and having found no game, approached them from the rear. He caught his foot in a vine, so Herbert said, and fell. His shotgun discharged. The heavy load at close range went through the lad's body. He died as the two men carried him out of the forest to their car.

Eva shed no tear. As one in a trance, she lay and looked without seeing. There are problems with which the mind of man can never deal. There is grief so keen that not even the corrosive action of time can dull it and make it bearable. I tried to comfort her, but my words must have carried little conviction. Only one statement made any impression. Its nature shows the extent of my search. It also shows the blackness of her despair. It was that her son was safe, that he would never suffer as she was suffering then.

There was an insurance investigation. The money finally was paid to Herbert. He would not contribute one dollar toward the boy's funeral expenses nor would he buy a marker for his grave.

The blight that always follows such a tragedy now began to settle. The old grandfather, at whose place the tragedy had occurred, died broken-hearted. Those other two who had been directly involved had their short day, withered, and passed away. One year after the boy's death, the man who had fired the fatal shot sent a bullet through his own brain. Not long afterwards Herbert developed heart trouble and came down upon his deathbed.

Of all the principal characters who had taken part in that frightful drama, only Eva remained. She drew further and further from those scenes—from those strange, wild dreams we call reality; but which in truth are as shadowy as her hope, faith, and love had been. Her almost superhuman courage was not enough and now faded. Isolated at last, hopeless, her feet were upon a path that wound through forgetfulness. From town to town, she drifted. Word of her came to me occasionally and then less and less often until she finally dropped from my mind.

Eighteen long years had passed since that fateful day. As I came to the end of my musings, I realized that Eva was waiting while I sat and held her card. I rang for my secretary to bring her in.

Eva's carriage was so erect, her poise so absolute, her personality so quiet and great that I stood motionless for a moment and looked at her in ill-concealed amazement. How had she come through all those years unbroken? Her face was smooth and fair. Except for the development of that strange and remarkable personality that hung like an aura about her, it was as if time had stood still. There was something of the unreal about her, as if she belonged not to this world. Her quiet gaze both interested and puzzled me. She apparently had obtained the tranquility of mind that so many of us long for but never find. Long before, I had reluctantly come to the conclusion that each mind is ever filled with worries and drifting, conflicting currents of dark thoughts, that this is a function of life and that calmness settles on mind and countenance only when life has passed. Yet, now before me was one who seemed to set this hopeless view aside.

Eva talked about her life in a manner as detached as if she were relating the history of another. Without the slightest reserve she told of scenes and incidents that gave me a pang of sympathy. As she continued in her flat monotone, I became aware that she knew little of the great world events that had taken place since the day of her son's death. No subject that I advanced brought any real response. Beneath the surface I began to see the outline of one whom long had walked in the glare of a tragedy—a glare so lurid that all else had paled into insignificance.

Soon she finished her simple account of the happenings of those years since I had seen her last. She sat motionless now, surrounded by that strange aura.

There is something familiar about it—but what? I wondered, while with contracted brow I peered at her.

Ah now! At last, I saw it—the extent of havoc wrought by that discharging gun. Those others were not the only ones to lose their lives. Her life also, as it had been, ceased that day.

And that mask-like countenance—I knew now what it meant; I had seen it oft before. Her face, without line or emotion, held the calm that lies upon the face of the dead.

The Woman with the Yellow Hair

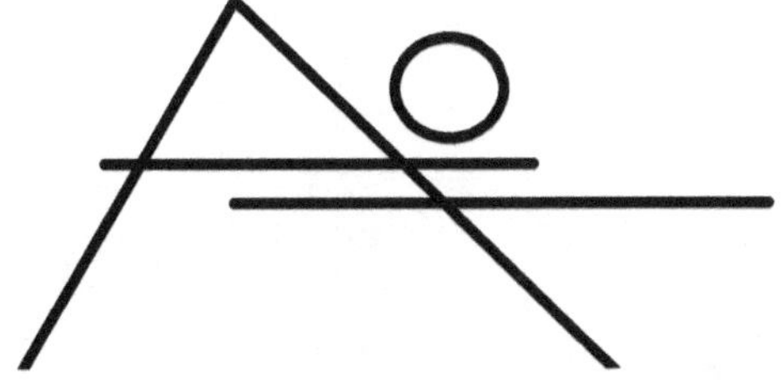

The Woman with the Yellow Hair

[Note: This fictional story, penned by the author as a young man, is included here to complete the collection.]

In my childhood, death was looked upon very differently from the way it is regarded now. Those were the years in which an age of morbid sentimentalism was slowly drawing to an end. It was an age of framed pictures, of weeping willows and tombstones, although not on the walls of my own home, upon the walls of many homes I entered; an age when flowers which had been laid on graves were mournfully picked up again, preserved in alcohol, placed under glass, and given a prominent place in the parlor as an ever-present reminder of death's visitation. It was the age of black coffins and black clothes of mourning, of funerals in which the minister preached loved ones saved or lost. It was an age in which most of the literature written and read was filled with gloom and forebodings.

Is it any wonder that in such surroundings a child, tender and impressionable, should come to look upon death not as the simple, natural cessation of the marvelous process of life; but that of an arch villain—one most real, inevitable, and terrifying? How well I remember the day I first realized that for those I loved and for myself there was no escape! Many a year has passed since that day. Observation and reason have gently soothed me and have covered those old feelings—just how deeply I do not know but deeply enough, it would seem, to carry me through.

Some misgivings on that score arise, however, when I remember how recent have been those morbid concepts. They were still uppermost in my mind when as a medical student I entered the dissecting hall.

Among my papers is a story, fiction in contrivance and plot, but grim reality in atmosphere and in regard to my own feeling. It was written shortly after the completion of my course in medicine while the recollections of those days were still fresh in my mind. As an example of the product of a mind which has not found itself, of a mind overwrought when suddenly placed in surroundings which it has always regarded with dread, I bring the story from the place where it has lain so long and record it for you here.

It all began as in the darkness I stood upon the stoop at the dissecting hall. My knocking on the door caused a muffled, booming sound that increased my uneasiness. There was no answer and, almost thankfully, I started to turn away when I heard the hollow tread of distant footsteps. Several moments passed as a clanking noise from within told me that the bolts were being drawn. The heavy door swung open. A peculiar odor, such as I had never smelled before, poured out and the form of a tall, thin, sinewy man with a lamp in this hand stood framed in the opening of the dissecting hall door.

"Is this Dr. Grimes?" I asked.

"Yes," he replied in a voice at once musical and metallic.

I introduced myself and told him the reason for my visit—that it was my first day at the medical school; that the sight of a dead body had always terrified me beyond words and for long afterwards would leave me dumb and thoughtful; that a misgiving had arisen as to whether I could, after all, put my fear aside and enter into the dread study of anatomy. I told how these gloomy thoughts had filled my mind all day and how my apprehension as to what my conduct would be on the morrow when the dissecting was to begin had hourly increased; and so it was that, seeing his light, I had resolved to come to the dissecting hall that very night and try to accustom myself to the sights which I knew lay before me.

He laughed without mirth. "All right," he said, "Come in."

He led the way into the great, dark hall. The flickering, uncertain light of his lamp shown over the rows of stark bodies laid out on the stone tops of the dissecting tables. A sensation of lightness came to my head and swept like a wave downward to my feet. I felt as light as a feather. This sensation passed in a moment, only to be followed by a strange numbness as I felt my kinship to those cold forms. In the deathly stillness I could hear the beating of my own heart.

It's the only difference, I thought. A pause and I shall forever join them in their silence.

At last, I raised my eyes. They could not carry to the corners of the room. The gray shapes of the small windows were discernible, but no light came through them. Creosote and other chemicals masked a sickening, pungent odor.

My guide was regarding me curiously and seemed to have read my every thought.

"Enough?" he asked, and as I could not answer, "Suppose we have a look at the vat where the bodies are preserved and kept."

He led me along the aisle, through a hallway, and down the steps into a large stone chamber. The air was heavy and stagnant and rank. The stone slabs of the floor were slippery from a thick, oily fluid.

It has been dripping on them all day as the bodies were drawn out of the vat, I thought.

The boards of the cover were piled to one side, and a great opening filled with the black, murky fluid yawned in the floor.

"Have a care," Dr. Grimes said. His voice echoed and reverberated about the room as he led the way along a slippery, narrow ledge beside the vat and threw open another door.

In this room stood a table-like machine. The top was placed on rollers and cogs. At one end, steel guides carried a long, thin saw.

"What is it?" I asked hoarsely.

"It is an apparatus with which to prepare cross sections for our final examination," he replied. "I made it myself. The table is calibrated. A cadaver is frozen and fastened to it, and the cross sections can be cut.

"That is the icehouse door," he continued, "and this one leads to the outside. After tomorrow all doors will be unlocked, and you may come and go as you please."

We retraced our steps and on the main floor entered a small study. There was a table in the middle of the room. On it, being dissected, were the remains of what had once been a human being. Dr. Grimes placed the lamp on a high stool and, seating himself, motioned me to a chair.

"There is an inherent dread of the dead in every living soul," he said. "Even those who do not fear death fear the dead. When I came here as a student and for many years thereafter, I felt as you do, but now I never think of it. In fact, this fall I have moved into a room adjoining this study in order that I may be near my work. I am carrying out a series of dissections to determine the variations of the chief nerve plexus. You may stay with me as long as you like."

As he bent over the body with the light of the lamp full upon him, I was able to observe at my leisure the face of my future instructor. He was a man of middle life. His general aspect was dark and gaunt—the pallor of his face, cadaverous. Jet black hair was matted about his receding forehead. His eyes were large and black and in them burned a strange intensity. His deft fingers moved swiftly in his dissection, and after a few moments I could see that he had become oblivious to my presence.

For a long time I sat, not daring to disturb him, until finally the strangeness of it all overcame me, and I said that I would go. He looked up with a start, asked me to remain a few minutes longer, and continued his dissection. After a while he looked at me thoughtfully, put down his knife, took up the lamp, and led me through the great hall to the door. I stumbled rapidly up the black path. At the top of the hill, I looked back. All was dark save the feeble yellow light in the window of his study.

Sixty students presented themselves at the dissecting hall the next morning. I was surprised to see a woman among them. She was in her early twenties and her fresh, young face and yellow hair lifted my thoughts out of the gloom into which they had sunk when I entered the hall. I learned that her name was Mary Louise Lane.

There was an awed hush about the room as the students stood huddled together looking at the cadavers.

Despite what he said, the feeling extends to Dr. Grimes, I thought, as I saw him hesitant, apparently uneasy, and heard him brusquely assign a place to the girl. However, I learned later that his disturbance had not come from fear; it was only that he had bitterly opposed the admission of a woman to the class but had been overruled by the faculty.

Day after day we toiled at the dissection. Dr. Grimes knew anatomy as a master. Its study and its teaching were the passions of his life. His swift, capable hands could disclose in a few minutes what would have required hours if probed at by the rest of us. Doubtless because of my visit to him that first night, he seemed to take an especial interest in my progress. He was never too tired or too busy to help in the clearing up of a difficult point or to assist me in a tedious dissection. He was hardly less helpful to the other members of the class—to all, that is, except the girl. As time passed, his rude and unjust criticism of her work grew until it became unbearable, and a representative from the class reported the matter to the head of the department.

What happened between the professor and our instructor we never knew, but Dr. Grimes became silent and sullen. He began to leave the class more to itself. Mary Louise seemed to realize her presence was the cause of his neglect and now rarely dissected with the rest of us.

"I will not let the class suffer on my account," she answered when I said that we missed her. After a pause she then added, "It is harder to carry out that resolution than you might think. The fact that Dr. Grimes lives there doesn't help any either. I am even more afraid of him than I am of the nameless silence that inhabits the hall. I know he will not pass me no matter what I do, but I am determined to finish the cadaver."

In the daylight, when the rest of us dissected, the inherent dread of the place seemed to be divided and diluted in proportion to the number present. Another thing I noticed was that as the dissection progressed, as the surface was destroyed and the bodies were slowly dissolved into their component parts, into muscles and blood vessels and nerves and gradually lost the appearance of the body as a whole, our uneasiness became proportionately less. True it was that a very small fragment still carried with it some of the feeling of death, as I found when I took a bone to my room for study; but I say that as the dissection progressed, the terror seemed to lessen somewhat—that the sum of a cadaver's parts does not equal the whole.

At night, however, when Mary Louise did much of her dissecting in silence and alone, the fear was, she told me, intensified and concentrated. Most of the cadavers were wrapped in wet cloths to keep them pliable, but the forms of the bodies and the knowledge that they were there even when her eyes were glued on her work slowly unnerved her. She became so tense that at every sound she held her breath and peered into the darkness beyond the limit of the light. She listened to every mouse run. Her own dissection of the cadaver's muscles of expression would set her heart pounding as the wavering flame of the lamp caused a seeming change in the sardonic grin, which perplexed her and to which no answer could be read in the sightless orbits. So it was that her work became more and more crude and that Dr. Grimes' criticism of it became more severe.

I often saw Mary Louise come and go.

If it is terrible for me, how much more so for the girl? I thought.

I felt a keen sympathy for her and resolved to help her pass the course. Under the pretext of reviewing my work, but really to teach her what I could and to bear her company in those dread hours, I began to dissect and go over the structures with her.

Mary Louise seemed very grateful for my presence.

"If Dr. Grimes comes in at all," she said, "he stands and looks at my dissection as if he sees something beyond the mere form of the structures and so, upsets me all the more."

We usually had the hall to ourselves, for the instructor had ceased his dissections in the anteroom. During those last days of the course, he seemed highly nervous and unstrung. Sometimes when we thought that we were alone and had dissected for a couple of hours, he would come up from the room which contained the vat and walk rapidly and aimlessly about the hall and through the other rooms, apparently unaware of our presence.

Several times during the year Dr. Grimes asked me to help at the vat. As little as I liked to do so, I felt that I could not refuse. Once, I had taken up the long pole with the sharp hook on the end and was feeling about in the fluid for a cadaver when the end of the pole touched one. I took a firm hold with both hands, gave a jerk or two to set the hook and then pulled the body to the surface. It was the body of a little child. With a quick shove, I released it and felt for another.

Again, one day at the end of the term, Mary Louise and I were dissecting when we heard the jog trot of the old horse and the rattle of the spring wagon that brought the bodies to the hall. As we looked out of the window, the driver stopped the horse and slid the white pine box out of the wagon. It dropped heavily on one corner and fell full length to the earth. Dr. Grimes stepped out of the door and spoke a few words to the driver. Looking upward, he saw us and asked if I would help.

"Bring Miss Lane with you," he said, much to my surprise.

Mary Louise and I went down together. We dragged and pushed the box into the basement, and Dr. Grimes brought out an ax. He swung wide, low and upward. The blow struck a little low and, partly lifting the end, drove the box across the floor. He followed and swung again. This time the back of the ax struck the top boards directly on their ends and sent them splintering and flying into the air, and we looked down upon the form of a young woman with long, yellow hair.

"Good!" exclaimed the instructor. "She will be fine for the cross sections! You remember. I showed you the machine that first night."

Mary Louise gave a cry and put her hand to her heart. She was as white as the corpse. Dr. Grimes looked at her with a great intensity.

Then he laughed—long and harshly.

Is he utterly devoid of pity?, I asked myself.

"I am going to take Miss Lane home, but will return if you need me," I said.

"No," he replied, "good-bye."

As we reached the top of the stairs, we heard him laugh again.

A couple of days after this, the dissections were finished. I was surprised and also somewhat puzzled when the instructor approved Mary Louise's work without a word. There now remained only the final examination, the one on cross section anatomy, and then the course would be over.

On the night before the last examination, I chanced to pass the dissecting hall and, seeing that its lights were burning, thought that perhaps Mary Louise was reviewing for the final test; but when I went in, I found no living soul in the room. I made my way into the hall and, seeing lights below, started down the stairs, only to meet the instructor on the way up. He was pulling on his coat and seemed surprised and agitated at seeing me.

"I have been preparing the material for the test," he said. "Come into my study and let me show you how it will be conducted."

From a shelf he took a stack of drawings done by a former class.

"This is the type of work that I want," he explained. "Each student will have a cross section of the body and will make a full-size drawing of it in colors. All structures must be labeled and each section given the correct number to show its position in the body. To do this you must refer to a full-length tracing, which I shall hang on the wall. I have divided the tracing with horizontal lines and have numbered the sections, beginning from the feet."

"Shall I go down and help you prepare the material?" I asked.

"No-no, I have finished," he replied quickly, putting his hand on my arm.

The Woman with the Yellow Hair

I bade him good night and made my way through the hall. That old feeling of dread had returned. A short way up the path I turned and looked back. There was something about the way the dismal, low building crouched under the great trees at the foot of the hill that completely unnerved me for a moment.

It is only that I associate its long use with the structure itself, I thought as I looked at its crumbling brick wall, almost devoid of windows, at its decaying shingle roof, and at its high, blackened smokestack. The dampness from the overhanging branches and the weeds that grew to the very wall, together with the peculiar odor that pervaded the atmosphere, gave the whole place a most unwholesome air. I looked at the faint light in the instructor's study.

How can a man live there and remain sane? I wondered. "Thank heavens! Another day, and I shall have finished with it all!"

It was very dark that bleak December night when the members of the class made their way toward the great hall for the final examination. As I entered, it was with a sense of relief that I noticed the cadavers had been removed and cremated. At each student's place was a thin cross section.

These frozen slices bore no resemblance to and scarcely suggested that they had been cut from a human body.

And yet it is there, I thought as I looked at my piece.

The roll was called. At the name of Miss Lane, the instructor hesitated and waited an instant, but there was no answer and he went on to the next. I looked at her vacant seat and saw that a cross section had been put out for her.

Dr. Grimes explained to the class the method of the examination.

"I have some work to do in my room, but will return before you have finished," he said, and then he departed.

We bent to our labors. We were so well trained in anatomical drawing that that part of the test passed quickly. The labeling of the structures severely tested our knowledge, however, for we were seeing them from a new angle; but even this was not as difficult as giving each section its correct number. Without comparing the slices, it was almost impossible to say whether a given section fitted into a certain place or should go an inch above or below it.

I was among the first to finish. As I sat and looked about the room, the same feeling of fear that I had always had came over me. While listening to the driving sleet against the windowpanes, I peered into the dark recesses of the room, at the tables that had carried their dread burden for so many years. I could see that the others were troubled by the same thoughts that troubled me.

At last, all were through and sat about the room in silence or whispered a few awed words to those nearest them. Presently someone suggested that we match the pieces together and reconstruct the body. It struck us all as a novel idea—something with which to occupy ourselves until the instructor returned. A space was cleared in the center of the room and a table placed there.

"Let's have number one," the leader called, and the student having the soles of the feet brought them forward.

Numbers two and three were added. Sometimes when a number was called, more than one student came forward, and the frozen sections had to be fitted and tried to see who was right. We included the piece from the unoccupied table.

As the form grew, fear and terror increased. Finally, when the last piece was placed, all shrank to the walls of the room in unspeakable horror, their eyes fixed upon the cadaver. It was the body of Mary Louise. I held to a table to keep from falling as I gazed at the form beneath the flickering light. A sickly pain gripped my heart.

There was a movement at the end of the hall, and we turned to see Dr. Grimes in the door. A wild light was in his eyes. He broke into a laugh, which rose higher and higher until it became a shrill, piercing shriek. He turned and ran.

"He is mad!" someone cried. "Seize him!"

With a concerted movement the entire class rushed after him. Down the dark stairs we pressed, into the dimly lit chamber below. With another wild shriek the instructor rushed along the narrow ledge. He slipped, and with a terrific impact his head struck the stone floor. For an instant he struggled on the brink and then plunged into the murky liquid of the vat.

We stood still but he did not rise. A moment afterwards, as of one accord, with the terror of the dead upon us, we turned and fled up the stairs, past the still white form, and out into the night.

The Last Word

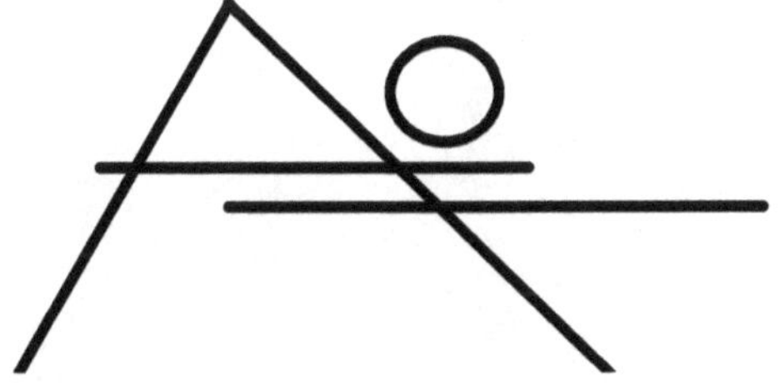

The Last Word

Petty pride leads to a fall. It is doubly dangerous in the practice of medicine. Here if anywhere, for the doctor's peace of mind as well as for the patient's welfare, it is essential to view each case objectively. To feel a little puffed up and give an overly optimistic prognosis based on the satisfaction of having well performed a difficult operation is to court disaster. For a doctor to hint that the medicine he prescribed was what cured a patient may lead to the patient's statement that he did not take the pills, but instead, threw them out with the trash. To seek the last word is often to lose any gain one may have made. In short, a good rule for the doctor is to "tend to his knitting" and let well enough alone. I received many lessons of this kind. A very pretty young woman gave one in particular to me.

When Madge Kennedy first came to me, she was sick. Anyone could see that at half a glance. Her slight form, wrapped in a soft green housecoat, slumped in the chair. Her auburn hair was disheveled, her face pale with suffering. Two years before, when she was twenty-one, she had undergone, so she said, an operation for a ruptured appendix. She had suffered pain off and on ever since. Lately the pain had become much worse. It was now unbearable.

Although I could see that her husband was deeply concerned, he did not enter into the conversation. He was several years older than his wife though in some ways not as mature. He seemed more like a curly-haired, overgrown boy than the able automobile mechanic I knew him to be. He was a tall man, supple but very strong. He had always been a happy-go-lucky fellow, but now that his luck was out, he was anything but merry. He kept wrinkling up his thin, aquiline nose as if he were about to burst into tears. In fact, there was a trace of moisture in those dark gray eyes. I was drawn to him, not only because of the friendliness and simplicity of his nature, but also because I was touched by the unusual degree of devotion he bore his wife. All during Madge's stay in the hospital, her husband hung around the place, brought in little presents, and kept her room bright with flowers.

During Madge's operation a great many adhesions were found and divided. So many in fact, that I had some uneasiness about her future and thus, when she pressed me for a prognosis, spoke somewhat reservedly. My manner caused her much anxiety which later reassurance could not quite overcome.

Sure enough! In six months' time she was back, this time dangerously ill with an acute intestinal obstruction. Again, she was operated upon, but imagine my relief when I found that her trouble was caused by a solitary, thread-like adhesion. This was removed, and I had the great satisfaction of telling her that she could forget doctors and hospitals—that her troubles were over. This statement proved to be far from true. To begin with, she did not believe it. She looked searchingly at me and asked if I were sure. When I was forced to hedge somewhat, her face fell.

Only a few days passed before Madge's husband brought her in again, bent double and complaining of great pain. She was put to bed and examined. In spite of what she said, it didn't take long to see that there was no real sign of trouble, nor was there enough evidence to convince me that she had any pain. She was kept under observation a day or two and then discharged. Madge left smiling. I thought I was through with her; but soon she returned, this time alone. Again, she was admitted for observation, examined, told that there was nothing the matter, and sent home. Back she came, again and again, each time complaining of severe pain. Knowing her former trouble, each time I had to consider her symptoms carefully. At times, when I would tell her that there was nothing the matter, she would seem satisfied; again, she would cry with pain until she was admitted to the hospital.

A day came when a new idea was injected into the picture. The head nurse reported to me that Madge ordinarily seemed happy and free of symptoms, but that as soon as her husband came on one of his now infrequent visits, she complained of pain greater than she could bear.

The management of the case was temporarily shifted to a psychiatrist who questioned both Madge and her husband. Both declared they loved each other dearly. Nothing was uncovered which could account for the woman's strange behavior. Sometimes when she would come to me, the symptoms that she described were so vivid I was almost persuaded that they were real, but always there was lacking some essential detail. She was merely remembering and reciting her old symptoms.

Soon now there began to be unmistakable evidence of trouble at Madge's home—something for her to cry about. Once when she came in, one of her eyes had a dark bruise beneath it.

"I ran into a door," she said.

She begged, wept, and complained of such pain that she was finally admitted. Upon examination, nothing new was found save dark bruises over her body. She rapidly improved and in a couple of days her mood lightened. Her husband came to see her. He was grinning and silent. Madge complained as long as her husband remained in the room.

I heard from a welfare worker who lived in the same village with them that at home Madge grunted and groaned until her husband was almost distraught; that whereas he had always been temperate, he now drank heavily and had begun to stay away from home at night.

"I can't say I blame him much," my informer added. "If I had to put up with that woman, there's no telling what I'd do."

All of this I discussed with the wife. She was told of the danger to her home, how her actions were destroying her husband and herself, that there was nothing the matter with her, and that if she did not believe me, she should go to some other doctor. I also reminded her of her husband's former kindness and advised her to try to keep from worrying him.

"Go to see your pastor," I suggested.

"I reckon I know when I hurt," she curtly told me.

The next day, as she was being discharged, I again gave her the same advice. Not a week had passed before she came back to the hospital. This time she was refused admission. She was furious.

A few days later, through the grapevine I heard the details of that dreadful night and the days that followed. At home Madge raved like one possessed. Her husband, having stood it as long as he could, left the house. Upon his return he found his wife lying in a pool of blood from a severed artery in her wrist. He called a local doctor, and when she refused treatment, she was forcibly held while the self-inflicted wound was sutured. As she continued to struggle and to make threats against her own life, the doctor declared her insane. A deputy sheriff was summoned and Madge was taken to the county jail. In no way tamed, she spent the next few days tugging at the bars of her cell, screaming and weeping. She refused to eat and had to be fed by force. When arrangements were complete for her admission to the asylum and the officers started to move her, she fought like a tiger, tooth and nail. It took several men to handcuff her and drag her to a car.

Despondent, confused, hopeless, unhappy with the lot fate had dealt her, dissatisfied with her husband and the little home he had been able to provide, and bitter against the doctors who would not take her word for the terrible pain she felt, Madge was driven to the state institution for the insane. The car stopped at the great iron gates. She scarcely looked at the forbidding, smoke-stained buildings. Anything would be better than what she had suffered, she felt.

Almost in a trance, she was checked in, searched, and taken to a doctor's office for examination, after which she was assigned to a ward. There she was dressed in the regulation blue denim worn by the inmates and was then taken by a nurse to a large sun porch off the hall.

Madge glanced into the bay and hung back. She received an authoritative shove.

"It was like a plunge into a pool of icy water," she told me later.

One look at that great, almost bare space; at the dingy walls and benches; at the windows with their heavy steel gratings; at the strange women standing there—women with a strange light in their eyes, huddled together, whispering to one another, eyeing her suspiciously—one look, and Madge's mind became clear. She realized how mixed up she had been and what she had given up. The image of her once pleasant little home floated before her, along with the vivid coloring of the hollyhocks she and her husband had planted.

From an adjoining building a scream broke in—long, piercing, weird, and unearthly. Again, the scream came. It froze her very blood. It came to its end.

Once more it began. Suddenly, smothered at its highest note, it stopped. There was silence.

Madge recovered in time to spring from the path of a heavy-set woman who waded past barefooted, with her shoes tied together by their laces and thrown over one shoulder and her skirt held high above her knees. Upon the woman's face fear was written—stark fear, as her eyes anxiously searched for something, turning first in one direction and then another. Madge looked on in horror as the woman reached the end of the hall, wheeled, and started back across the floor.

"Oh Doctor!" Madge cried as the physician who had just admitted her passed at the other end of the hall.

She ran to him. "Oh Doctor, let me go home. This is all a dreadful mistake. It is some terrible dream."

"Now don't you worry, little girl," the old doctor told her kindly. "Soon you will get used to it. Everything will be all right."

"No, Doctor," she pled. "Listen to me please. I wouldn't talk to you when I came but I will now. I know I have been a fool, but I don't belong here. Please examine me again and let me go."

The doctor looked long at her and then took her with him into his office. He talked with her at length and when he had finished sat and tapped his desk with a pencil. Finally, without a word to Madge, he told a nurse to take her back to the sun porch.

As they approached a turn in the hall, Madge heard a peculiar sound as if of escaping steam—S-S-S-S-S. There was a pause, and then she heard it again. She rounded the corner and froze. Before her was a teapot—a teapot in the flesh, yet as rigid as if cast from clay—clay to which The Potter had failed to add that all-important spark. It was a thin, gray-haired old woman. Her left arm, akimbo, formed the handle; her right, held upward and outward, the spout. S-S-S-S-S, she went with each long expiration—S-S-S-S-S. The nurse took Madge's arm and led her past to her own group.

Now she heard the sound of a distant voice singing somewhere on the grounds. Nearer it came, and through the window she saw the form of a woman hurrying by. The woman was singing at the top of her lungs

"I'm forever blowing bubbles, pretty bubbles in the air."[4]

The song grew fainter and was lost.

"What does it mean?" Madge asked.

After some hesitation on the nurse's part, she was told that the woman's husband and three children had been killed in a wreck. "Bubbles," they called the woman.

Madge turned her attention to the strange sights close about her. She repulsed the advances of those inmates who came to tell of their delusions and to ask if she could hear the nonexistent voices that were so real to them. Try as she might, she could not take her eyes from the wader. With her heart in her throat, Madge watched the woman's ceaseless and pathetic search for solid ground upon which to rebuild her life. As she watched, she thought of the way the earth had slipped from beneath her own feet.

The day wore out. Madge begged the attendants to lock her up by herself. She was terrified as her mind exaggerated the dangers of the night. Finally, she was assigned to a little room, and thankfully, she heard the key turn.

Through long, black hours she lay awake, her hands clamped to her ears; but they could not shut out the sound of running feet, the shouts, and the cry of "Dogs!"

"Kill that dog over there, kill that dog over there, kill that dog over there," cried a strange, unearthly voice. Again, and again the cry broke through Madge's barrier. "Kill that dog over

---

4. Jaan Kenbrovin and John William Kellette, "I'm Forever Blowing Bubbles," (Jerome H. Remick and Co., 1919), accessed Oct. 24, 2021, https://american history.si.edu/ collections/search/object/nmah.

there, kill that dog over there," until finally exhausted, she fell asleep.

The next day Madge refused to leave her cell. There was a long argument. In the end she was allowed to have her way. She wanted no food, but under threat of forced feeding ate a little. Some magazines were brought for her, but she could not turn a leaf. Her best efforts could not shut out the sound of that ceaseless, terrible laughter that floated up to her, could only muffle somewhat the interminable rattling as hour after hour some inmate of an adjoining building shook the steel grating of his window, could not shut out Bubbles. All day the song rang in Madge's ears as the singer, in her furious restlessness, roamed among the trees.

A day passed, and another, and another. They were all alike—all like some horrible, hopeless nightmare—until one afternoon a week after Madge had come. The door opened and a nurse brought in Madge's pretty clothes and told her that her husband was waiting with a car to take her home.

It was three months later that she and her husband came to see me. It was hard to believe she was the same girl. I looked at her with a certain delight in her vitality and youth. Madge was a slender, graceful, auburn-haired beauty. Her smart, stylish dress, and high-heeled pumps matched her green eyes. They also told me how most of her husband's wages were spent. Her eyes and teeth were sparkling. She seemed so healthy, so happy. Her husband, now again proud of his property, was broadly grinning.

"The last three months would have been the happiest of my life if it hadn't been for the dreams at night." Madge said. She hesitated a moment and then added, "I expect they have been anyway, even with that."

"Well, now forget it," I said. "It was a terrible remedy, but it is over and past. There is nothing to regret. It took that to cure you."

"Huh! Cure me?" she queried, stiffening.

"Yes," I replied, a little taken aback.

She looked at me long and appraisingly. Perhaps she read in my face a glimpse of a now rapidly fading overconfidence in the position I had taken, that certain I-told-you-so-all-the-time-ness. If so, she didn't see it long. I came down to earth at the tone of her very first word.

"No," she coolly replied, "It didn't cure me. I just made up my mind I'd never say anything about it no matter how I hurt."

The Detour

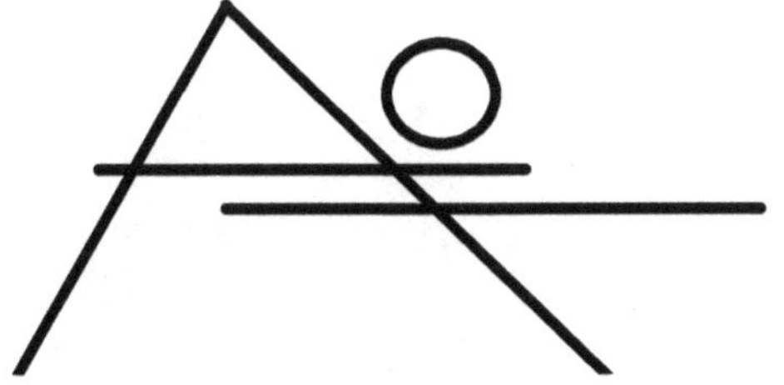

The Detour

When I first saw Nellie Morrison, I was a teen-aged boy. When I saw her again, I was a mature, practicing surgeon. Thus, the beginning and the end of her story are from my personal knowledge. The rest I patched together from bits told me through one long, dark night.

A little girl walked toward me down the cool wagon road through the woods. She was singing a soft but joyous song and swinging her sunbonnet by its strings. The splotchy pattern of light and shade played upon her freshly starched dress. There was a flash of gold in her hair at the moment the sun struck it. Her blue eyes were smiling, and the springtime of life was in her cheeks and lips.

I shall not tire you with an account of how Nellie lost her parents and their property. Suffice it to say that these sorrows did but make her more gentle and thoughtful. In her loneliness, she fell in love with a young mill hand that visited the neighborhood; thus, her sixteenth birthday found her married and, like a transplanted wildflower, living in a dingy house near the mill.

That first bleak day, Nellie stood a long time and looked at the small, dilapidated house that was to be her home. Dingy from soot, it sat perched on stakes above the sloping yard of clay and cinders. She turned to the mill below. Its great stack was belching forth a cloud of smoke.

"What are you thinking about?" her husband asked, regarding her curiously.

"I am wondering how many people have come here just starting out like we are and what has become of them," she replied. A moment later she had found herself.   "It is   the only home we can provide for the children that we want, and we will make the most of it; but we will not live here always, will we, Fred? I want the country for them like I had."

"No," he replied simply.

So, their life at the mill began. They had little money, but there was little required. A few iron and tin kitchen utensils, a bed and its covering, a few splint-bottomed chairs, a lamp, a table, and a rag rug for the hearth—these, together with her energy, cleanliness, and care were enough to furnish the house. Mixed with that indefinable touch of a woman's hand, they made of the house a home.

Nellie was very tired when that first night came, but she felt a sense of satisfaction at their progress. Before going to bed, she went out on the porch to see the stars. None shone through the cloud of smoke. She watched instead, the sparks of the stack and the rows of lights in the windows at the mill.

The next morning Nellie awoke with a cry and wild pounding of the heart. It was quite dark. A shrill, piercing noise filled the room. Every moment it gained in intensity. The very house vibrated.

"What is it?" she whispered, trembling.

"It's the whistle. It's time to get up."

The sound slowly died away and then began once more. Fred lit the lamp.

"Why, what's the matter? You look so white," he said.

"It startled me so. Does it blow every morning?" she asked with a sinking of her heart.

"Why, of course," Fred replied. "The sound of the whistle is the first thing I can remember."

Those early days filled with their cares, passed rapidly. The interior of the house grew brighter and more cheerful. Gradually Nellie added ruffled gingham curtains to the windows, yellow oilcloth with scalloped edges for the shelves, an embroidered sheath to hold the twisted lamp lighters, and other things which she found time to make. How warm and safe it seemed within when the window shutters were closed and fastened and the door was secured with a heavy bar against the winter night! The small, open fire cast its flickering shadows over the room.

Nellie knitted and looked into the fire, her soul at peace, dreaming of another spring more wonderful than all that had gone before. By closing the door, she could shut the mill out. It was the whistle that unnerved her. Its harsh blast never failed to leave her white and trembling with a fear of something—she knew not what.

"I shall get used to it," she told herself many times, but it was always the same.

Spring came at last. With a thought of her old home, Nellie slipped away to the bank of the river, the one lovely spot near the town. The overcast skies of winter had become a soft, thin blue, and every bud in the forest had begun to swell with the irresistible tide of life. She was standing in a meadow watching the fresh, young grass and the tender, yellow leaves of the willow when she felt the first stir of new life within herself. Child that she was, she was overcome with wonder and delight.

Her husband received the news with little comment. He began a crude cradle and by working on it each night soon finished it. With loving care Nellie lined and decorated it. How eagerly and tenderly did she cut up her own clothes to reform them to a smaller mold!

When her baby was born and she held his warm, soft body in her arms and satisfied herself that he was perfectly formed, it seemed as if all her longings had been fulfilled, and life in its richness would now unroll before her. These were days when she held him close to her and dreamed. It was only when she heard the shrill blast of the whistle or looked out upon the mill that her heart would falter.

"We must save, I can't let my baby grow up here," she would think.

The years passed—many, too many of them. A morning came when Nellie filled two dinner pails and with other children about her and yet another baby in her arms, stood and watched her oldest son walk with his father toward the mill. His coarse clothes were transparent to those eyes that saw only his childlike body, his slender limbs, the close-cropped flaxen hair, and the deep groove down the back of his thin neck.

It won't be long, Nellie thought as she entered the house to calculate her savings. Soon he can go off to school.

Another winter came and went, and the breath of still another was in the air. Times were hard. Fred's wages were cut, their savings spent. Another child, a tender girl, went into the mill. Nellie cried herself to sleep that night.

"I will never bear another child to go into the mill, I can't! I can't!" she sobbed.

Nellie was tired. Every hour was filled with anxiety for the safety of her children in the mill. The house was increasingly hard to keep clean with the soot forever settling on the windows and the mud and cinders forever being tracked in from the alley by many little feet. The furniture was old and shabby now as the accumulation of cots and clothes and plunder littered the place. There was no time to attempt to beautify it. The geraniums and nasturtiums, which for a while had distinguished their yard from the other yards of the alley, had perished long ago.

Nellie's strength was failing. She had fallen behind in her work. Though she was the first one up in the morning and the last to go to bed at night, the long, weary day was not long enough in which to complete her tasks. She never had a single day of rest. Her life had become a monotonous life of toil. The brief periods of sorrow and pleasure that came did nothing to lessen the tedium of her existence.

Though thankful that her husband and children had work, she felt in a vague, indefinite way that their wages had been calculated to give the bare necessities of life, with a small surplus out of which she was to raise as many workers for the mill as possible. The weekly paycheck was spent at the company's store before it was earned. Once she had contemplated the future of her little girls, planning and wondering how she could save them from a life like her own; but the hopelessness of it all had discouraged such thoughts and she had ceased to have them. She had forgotten the bend in the placid river that she once loved to visit. This fall, while she was on an errand, her path lay again by its brim. She gave it no thought. She did not raise her eyes to the steep bluff on the opposite side where the red and brown and yellow leaves were touched and made glorious by the rays of the sinking sun.

Nellie had become nervous and sleepless. She would start up only to find that the whistle had not blown. Sometimes during a storm at night, as she slowly regained consciousness, at that moment when the kinship of sleep and death is so apparent, she would feel that the mighty roaring in her ears was the roaring of the wind and the beating of the rain on her own grave.

It was still black night as Nellie lay and listened to the whistle of the mill. Its low tone grew shriller, louder, and more and more insistent until the very earth seemed to vibrate and tremble. The uproar slowly receded to a mere moan and had all but died away when it commenced once more. Again, and again it rose and fell. To her it was the cry of some great monster making its demands for the human life that must be fed into its maw that day, and she cried aloud as she thought that it was lying in wait for her own flesh and blood as yet unborn.

For a week she had been nervous and heartsick. The old symptoms were upon her. She had hoped against hope that she was mistaken, but every day increased her certainty that she must again bring a child into the world.

The whistle grew fainter and ceased altogether. She continued to listen. At first the silence was as disturbing as the noise had been. After a few moments, it too became less intense.

"O God, I can't go through that again!" she sobbed. "I'll die! I'll go raving crazy!"

She was aroused by her husband's voice reminding her that it was time to cook breakfast.

After Fred and the older children had gone to the mill, Nellie washed, dressed, and fed the younger ones. More than ever before she noticed their pale, thin forms and their threadbare clothes. She reeled with faintness as she went into the kitchen to wash the dishes. Weak and sick, she sat down in the corner. Her ears were ringing. Vaguely she thought of the whistle. All at once she saw a way of escape. She knew of other women in the village who had revolted at such a time and had opposed nature successfully. She had always considered such a practice a mortal sin and looked upon it with horror. Now she could excuse these women whom she had formerly condemned. She put on her hat and coat and walked to the home of a friend for whom she obtained the information necessary to carry her resolution into action.

All the next day she waited. Nothing happened. Doubts as to the wisdom and righteousness of her act rose to haunt her. In regret she realized that an act once done must stand through eternity. She prayed to God for his pardon and mercy and waited.

The following morning dawned clear and cold. She went about her work with a new and strange sensation of lightness and freedom. Her body seemed all at once to have become perfectly attuned to its environment. She felt neither warm nor cold. She did her work rapidly and without effort. For her every day was washday. After wringing out the garments, she started across the yard to hang them out. She noticed that it now seemed a great distance and that it took a long time to raise her foot and set it down again. The sun was dazzlingly bright, and flashes of light played before her eyes. She reached the clothesline and held to it. Suddenly she became conscious of a feeling of icy coldness. She was unaware of getting into bed and scarcely aware of the chill that shook her or of the great wave of heat that slowly spread over her body. The day dragged into a wearisome age of confusion and disconnected thoughts. Then her mind became clear. The terrible throbbing in her brain had passed.

It was late that night when her family physician called me to see her. In an hour's time I reached the town where she lived. Soon I stood by her bed and looked down upon her worn face. Although accustomed to seeing the mill women prematurely aged from labor and care, I was still unprepared for what I saw there.

"Thirty-eight," I repeated after her husband as I looked at the straggly gray hair, the thin, drawn, almost toothless mouth, and the worn hands with fingers still curved as if the implement they had been holding had just fallen from their grasp.

The resilience of life had left her bloodless cheeks. Moisture stood in the creases beside the nose. Her eyes and wrinkled skin were a dusky yellow color. About the whole bed was an air of dampness and cold as if it were a part of the winter night that the fire could not dispel. When I felt her pulseless wrist, I recognized another and more absolute chill that extended to her elbow and told me that she was beyond a doctor's aid.

I had given such stimulants as I could. While I stood looking down at her, she opened her eyes.

"You feel better now, don't you?" I asked.

She looked at me expectantly, and when she saw no sign of recognition in my eyes gave a sob and a little piteous cry.

"O Doctor, don't you know me? It's Nellie."

Nellie Morrison! Returning memories surged through my mind. I took her hand again, encouraged her all I could, and sat by her bed. Brokenly she spoke of the past until at last she was still.

For a long time, we remained in silence. Then a slight movement caused me to raise my head. I leaned over and closed her eyes. A moment later there arose a harsh, rumbling sound that became louder and shriller. It was the whistle, but it was not for her.

I gazed at her and beyond at a little country girl walking down the cool wagon road through the woods, swinging her sunbonnet by its strings. She paused at the bend of the road, looked back, waved her hand, and passed from sight.

The Monument

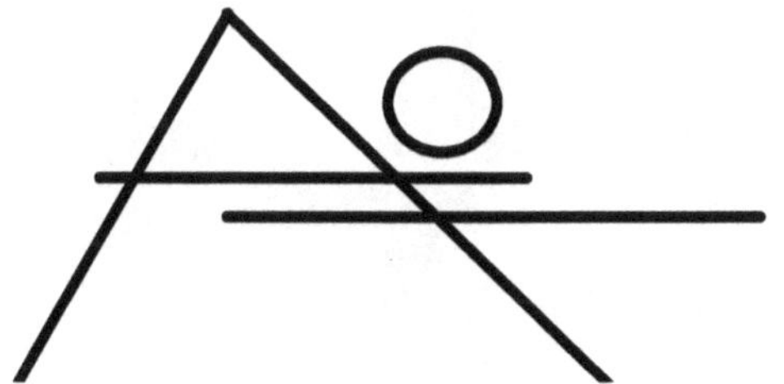

The Monument

> . . . the race is not to the swift, nor the battle to the strong, neither yet bread to the wise, not yet riches to men of understanding, nor yet favor to men of skill; but time and chance happeneth to them all.
>
> Ecclesiastes 9:11 (KJV)

No, those attributes that usually suffice are not always enough. They are not enough when a gathering storm arises from without a man's tiny sphere of influence, looms on the horizon, and, advancing, sweeps over him. Neither can one's utmost endeavors prevail against the legend on the die which chance occasionally casts down before him. Time and chance then—these two—are well known to us as causes of success and failure. They are accepted in our modern thought.

There is still another cause of disaster. There must be, for here nothing is left to chance. Its essence lies in that shadowy realm which no mind can penetrate. It is manifest in the series of events that follow when misfortune singles out its victim and, like some hound from hell, dogs his every step, camps upon his trail, frustrates him at every turn, jostles his hand at every important stroke, and never lets up, following him to his grave and yet beyond.

The ancient Greeks had an explanation for this too—one of the Furies. Though the decrees of their deities were considered inexorable, the Greeks, nevertheless, anxiously built magnificent temples in their honor, represented them in statues of surpassing beauty, and sacrificed to them the black sheep born to their flocks.

Today we do not subscribe to these old pagan beliefs, yet our minds, while refusing to accept them, fail utterly in an attempt to supply a rational substitute.

An instance of this kind of ill fortune once came to my attention. Its victim, strangely enough, was one whose family had long been associated with those old religions. His childhood home, he told me, had been in Crete. The very house in which he was born was built of stone pilfered from some ancient shrine.

"I gad, Doctor! I thought everything would be right in America, but no! It followed me!" said Timaeus Theotolamus, master marble cutter, who only recently had come to us as an immigrant. Disappointment and anxiety were evident in his rapid, high-pitched, foreign voice.

"It just wants you to feel at home, that's all," jokingly said the man who had come in with him from a nearby stone yard.

The injured man was young, not quite thirty. He was small but wiry and strong. I was struck at the contrast between his almost chalk-white skin and the blackness of his hair and eyes, a contrast extending into the short, black stubble which a daily shave could not keep down.

His accident, though painful, was nothing serious. The fingertips of one hand had been caught when Tim's assistant had suddenly slipped as the two were lowering a stone upon its base. After I had sutured and dressed the wounded fingers, I let him go.

The Monument

A day or two later, when he came in alone, I had more time to spend with him. He was good-natured, agreeable, and friendly. As we leisurely talked together, I asked the meaning of his strange anxiety. Little by little he told me that too many misfortunes had befallen him and that whether it was his fault or not, whether he used great care or not, he was always getting hurt. This started while he was an apprentice and had continued ever since. At first, he thought nothing of it; but as time passed and the accidents increased in frequency and severity, a feeling of impending doom had crept over him. He and his wife decided to leave everything they had ever known and start life afresh in the New World.

His phobia was too real to be laughed away and when I attempted to reason with him, I found this also was impossible. As he said, there was the record.

After this I didn't see him for a while. He had opened his own yard in another town. It wasn't too long, however, before he returned to his old job and after that to me. This time it was with a crushed foot.

At first Tim's misfortunes and fears were a cause of levity among his fellow workers and they teased him unmercifully.

"Well, you haven't seen any black cats today, have you?" they would ask.

However, as Tim's bad luck continued, the joking ceased. With each succeeding mishap Tim's dejection increased, seemingly out of all proportion to the importance of the injury.

Some of the men began to be afraid to work with him. More than one stonecutter left the yard—left with a feeling that a curse hung over it.

"Next time is the last," Tim said to me one day as I gave him first aid for a minor injury.

"Oh no!" I replied, in an attempt to reassure him "the Wheel of Fortune is due for a spin. Next time it will be someone else's number that will come up."

I was wrong. As I heard the tone of a voice over the telephone, I knew that Tim's prediction had been fulfilled. The caller urged me to come to the yard with all possible speed.

As I arrived, Tim's fellow workers had just succeeded in prizing up the great stone and dragging him from under it; they were now carrying him into a large, open shed.

There he looked up at me and in short gasps whispered, "It is over. It is all over," and then added, as a look of terror came into his eyes, "I hope."

There, a few minutes later, stretched out upon the clay floor and the granite spalls and dust, surrounded by the rough tools of his trade and by blocks of stone—some as they had come from the quarry, some partly cut, some already lettered for the graves they were to mark—there, among those ever-present reminders of the mortality of men, in those surroundings where Tim had lived his life, he laid it down.

Even after his wife had come and gone, even after his crushed body had been carried away, I stayed on among his friends at the yard. All were saddened and shocked. All were awed, as was I, that the accident, if it had to happen, should have singled out this man as its victim. There was something here we could not understand. All agreed that neither this mishap nor any of the others that had taken place over the years had been, strictly speaking, his fault. Yet he was the only one there who had ever received an injury.

"You don't suppose he could have been right after all?" one ventured. "He thought bad luck was out to get him."

"Bosh!" exclaimed another. "Don't tell me that he's got you to believing such tommyrot."

"I didn't say I believed it. I just wondered why everything had to happen to him."

"It didn't have to. That's all nonsense. This is the twentieth century. It wasn't anything but a streak of bad luck and the fact that he held such ideas as you are getting now. That's what killed him."

I was told the cause of the accident. A large monument was being loaded into a truck. As the stone was rolled up the skids, for some unaccountable reason, one of the beams slipped.

"Watch out!" rang the sharp, warning cry as the stone tilted.

It rocked back, tilted again, moved over slowly, and fell. The men who had been loading it stepped aside. Tim was lettering a stone in the shed. As the shout rang out, he dropped his tools, wheeled and in terror sprang from the safety of the shed directly into the path of the falling stone.

The men told stories of other misfortunes that had come to Tim, for his hard luck had not been limited to personal injuries.

A stonecutter who had worked in Tim's yard described in some detail the incident that finished his business venture. A successful and promising bid for the construction of a mausoleum was made, but in its building everything went wrong. Extras and accidents sapped away most of the expected profit. Finally, in spite of all misfortunes, the walls of the structure were completed and all was ready for the roof. To cut this, an enormous piece of stone eleven and a half feet by twelve and a half feet and nearly two feet thick was quarried. It was loaded upon an extremely strong, low-wheeled wagon and drawn from the quarry by four yokes of heavy oxen.

With great care and labor, the stone was cut to shape and polished. To raise it into its place, Tim, after advice from an engineer, erected a derrick. Its uprights were made of heart-locust posts twelve inches in diameter. A large chain fall was purchased, and a chain thought to be well able to carry the calculated weight was borrowed. The stone had been raised but a short distance when the chain parted. No one was hurt as the great slab fell, but a piece of granite a foot across came away from its corner.

Tim arranged for another contractor to complete the work, turned his little business over to his creditors, and returned to his former employment at the old yard.

The stories came to an end. After a long minute the silence was broken.

"Isn't all this some tale though!" a man exclaimed. "What could have been wrong?"

"Nothing," said the proponent of logic who had referred to the twentieth century. "Every one of these accidents can easily be explained."

"Yes, but that doesn't explain their number," answered the other.

"I knew something like this was going to happen. It bothered me until I couldn't half work," said a man who had not until now entered the conversation. "I got about as jumpy as Tim was."

The owner of the yard spoke again. "It's a wonder we weren't all killed," he said. "You couldn't talk Tim out of it. It had to be. Now maybe we can get this fog out of our heads."

The conversation shifted. A man told of Tim's kindness and consideration for everyone with whom he worked, of a very sizable favor Tim had once done for him when he was in dire need. As I left, yet another man was beginning another story of Tim's unselfishness.

A few days later the men at the stone yard declared their intention of erecting a memorial to Tim's memory—a stone that would compensate as far as was now possible for the misfortunes of his life.

"A stone that is a stone," one of the men said to me.

"No," the man replied when I suggested that all of Tim's friends be allowed to contribute, "we want to do it ourselves."

As a body, the men went to the quarry. With their experienced eyes they examined all the stones available and after some discussion, narrowed the choice to three or four large granite blocks of different sizes and shapes. To bring out any hidden flaw or seam they poured water over the stones still being considered and finally selected a beautiful and perfect one. It was a tablet-like shaft wider than a grave and would when finished and set upon its base extend to a height of over seven feet. Each of the men paid to the owner of the quarry an amount rather large for men in their circumstances, and the stone was moved to the yard.

Now the men set about deciding upon a design that would be suitable for their material. The drawing, which the stonecutters finally evolved for the pattern, was, as far as I could tell, entirely original. The extreme top of the stone was to be cut in a flattened version of the dome of a Moslem temple. They had this mixed in with Grecian architecture. At first, I felt somewhat dubious and disappointed; but over the months, as the work grew and as I saw it from time to time, I became almost enthusiastic. The delicate, restrained tracery up the edges, the very grandeur of the stone, and the sweep of the plane surface prepared for the inscription were enough to carry out the men's conception of the beautiful and, in reality, to make of the monument a noble thing.

Neither Rome nor Athens was built in a day, nor was this monument soon cut. Each holiday, each Saturday afternoon, at least some of the stonecutters came to work on the shaft. Gradually it took shape and one Fourth of July, after more than a year had passed, all hands brought their lunches and assembled to give the monument its finishing touches. Long afterwards one of those present told me what happened that day.

Under the shed, face up, across heavy wooden trusses rested the slab, ready for the inscription. Tim's wife had brought in a long middle name. When the full name was laid out, the letters seemed to the men to be small for a tablet of such height. Someone suggested that larger letters be used and the names placed step like across and down the face of the stone. There being present not only a quorum but also a full representation of those concerned, a vote was taken and the queer suggestion adopted then and there. Some of the men worked upon one part of the lettering and some upon other parts, and the inscription was all but finished by mid-afternoon of that hot, dry day.

"Watermel-o-o-n-s!" came the long, drawn out and welcome cry from a passing wagon. One man left his work and went down to the road. Presently he returned with a long, striped melon. The last letter was finished. A few old newspapers lying handy were spread upon the stone, and the juicy melon was placed upon them and cut.

The men sat here and there upon the edge of the stone. As they ate the melon, the talk fell upon that unfortunate man in whose memory the memorial was carved. They spoke of his affability, of his luckless life.

"He had it bad, didn't he?" said one of the stonecutters with a smile as he turned the mood of the gathering into a lighter vein. "A thing like that is all in the mind. I can't help believing he would have been all right if he hadn't kept so scared."

The conversation then turned to the monument. All agreed that it would be the finest in the cemetery. They reviewed the various steps that had been taken. It was the time for passing out compliments and claiming credit. Each called attention to any suggestion he had made to add to the beauty of the stone.

In high spirits one sang out, "And just to think! In spite of Tim's old jinx, we have finished this job without a single slip up."

All laughed. They arose, wiped their knives upon their overalls, and put them away. The rinds, scattered here and there upon the papers, were picked up and thrown out of the shed. The sodden, rotten newspapers tore as they were taken up. In pieces they were stripped up and cast to one side. With cupped hands the men swept the juice and seeds from the stone and began to dry it with old sacks.

A large splotch of stain, dark with a pink cast at the edges, covered the middle half of the face of the stone and dripped down its edges. There was as yet no sense that all was not as it should be, of the damage that had been wrought. Buckets of water were brought and thrown upon the stone. The stain was unaffected. Soap and warm water and a cloth were brought and used and when this failed, the men, with mounting uneasiness, tried detergents and a brush. Consternation was now written on every face. They tried everything they could think of. Everything made the stain worse. It was at length decided that further attempts to remove it would only carry it deeper and deeper into the pores of the stone. It was a gloomy and crestfallen group that sat down in council.

"Well, now what?" someone asked.

One man proposed that they buy another stone and start afresh. He brought up the fact that the idea behind the unusually handsome memorial was to try to compensate Tim for his luckless life, and to make up to him as far as they could for all the jokes they had poked at his fears.

"We can't stop now," he declared. "That would be to let him down—and us too."

"It would be one weary job," someone sighed.

A hush fell. The recollection of the cost involved and the time and labor that had been expended mitigated their grief somewhat, lessened their resolution, and spoke strongly against another attempt.

"Besides that," said a man whom the stain had converted to Tim's way of thinking. "If we tried once again or a dozen times, we couldn't cut a stone for him without ruining it."

"Let's put it up just as it is," said another with sudden inspiration. "It tells the story of his life better than would any words we could carve upon a stone. Let's put it up and say nothing about it."

Put it up they did.

Time has changed it little. Its distinguishing and significant feature is a large, irregular splotch. It is as if some outraged avenger has mixed a heavy, hellish brew and with it blotted out the name of that ill-fated man. A long drip from the blot, like an accusing finger, points downward toward his grave.

The Story of the Talents

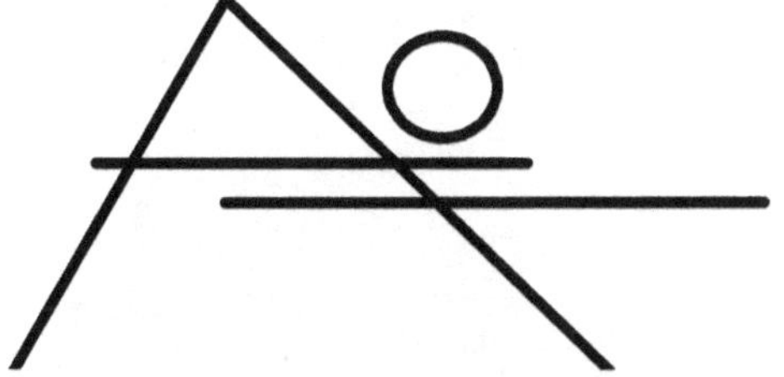

The Story of the Talents

In her little home at the edge of town, Maggie Lindoll lay dying. All about the house was a strange stillness, as if it too in some way realized that she was taking her departure; but through the open door the sun was streaming, a lark sang in the meadow, a soft wind murmured in the trees, and a mother hen with her brood came into sight, clucking and scratching in the loam beside the path. Across the road a man and a little boy in blue overalls were burning off a new ground. Like the advancing line of their fire with its sparks flying skyward, life was still going on, kindling a new blaze before it, while in the waste behind lay the ashes of the forms that for a while had supported and brought forward the flame.

As I sat in the hall and waited, my mind slowly carried me back to the day I had first seen Maggie. Out of the past the form of a young woman on a tall, bay horse rose before me. I saw again her sparkling, dark eyes, flushed cheeks, and smiling red lips. Her brown hair was blowing across her forehead, beneath the brim of a severe black hat, and her skirt was hanging full and long from her slender waist.

Maggie was the daughter of a well-to-do planter. At his death she and her older sister inherited his worldly goods. For several years Maggie traveled and studied abroad. Some talk of an unfortunate love affair drifted back, but no one ever knew its particulars. It was a quiet and serious Maggie who returned to live with her sister in the great house amid the oaks which had sheltered her family for generations.

My mind now swiftly followed her changing fortunes.

The two sisters had advanced into their forties and had become settled in that middle age which seems insusceptible of change, when the unexpected happened. Maggie fell in love with a man who worked on their plantation and married him in spite of the protests of her sister and friends. Their worst fears were soon justified. Her husband assumed charge of her inheritance and through reckless expenditure and unwise investments quickly dissipated it. When all but the last of her fortune was gone, he deserted her. Maggie was left alone on a little farm at the edge of town, with the necessity of wresting a living from its poor soil.

A short time afterwards her baby was born—a girl who was given her mother's name.

"I have wanted her all my life," Maggie said to me that day. "I didn't want to die without leaving a child."

The little girl was delicate and sickly. Many times, I saw the mother silent and anxious as she walked the floor with the baby in her arms. When the child was two years old, she had a serious illness and the care of nursing her was added to the work of the farm. There were days when the mother did not take off her clothes and had no rest save for a few minutes of fitful slumber on the edge of the child's bed. The night the crisis approached and life hung on a thread, I could not persuade Maggie to leave the bed where she sat watching the child's every breath and, even after I had assured her that the danger was past, for a long time she remained there in silence.

The Story of the Talents

This crisis proved to be the end of all the child's illnesses. She became robust and strong and in the spring, as I drove by, would wave to me from the field where her mother was at work.

One Christmas Eve when I had gone to leave the little girl a present, I sat by the fire and watched the mother fill a tiny stocking with walnuts from the farm and the candy, knitted mittens, and a rag doll which she had made.

"What is the greatest delight that you find in her?" I asked as I looked at the little worn shoes on the hearth. "Is it such a time as this?"

Maggie gazed into the fire. "Of course this is a delight," she replied, "and there is an interest and happiness in watching her develop day by day; but my real joy is in dreaming of the future, of the woman she will make. Did you ever see anyone so sweet and gentle? I have never seen her fret for what she could not have. Her little body is perfect—her eyes too—and the texture of her skin. I want to teach her to be self-reliant, to have no false pride, to stay as fresh and simple as she is now. I only wish my sister knew her. She would learn to love her as I do."

"Your sister has never come?" I asked.

"No," she replied.

Without the slightest shame Maggie went among her old friends to ask them for their sewing and other odd jobs. Many a time I saw her leading the little girl by the hand as she went from door to door with a basket of eggs or lettuce on her arm. Once, I chanced to be at a house when Maggie called for scraps of cloth with which to make rugs one half for the other. She wore a large garment of brown, which had the appearance of having been made from one of her husband's cast-off coats; her soft white hair and her pale face contrasted strangely with her rude clothes.

How nice the little girl looks, and how like her mother, I thought. She has the same straight, fine nose and delicate mouth; the same calm, dark eyes; the same carriage of the head.

There followed several years during which they had no serious illnesses and I neither saw nor thought of them often until that winter morning when little Maggie came to my office. She was fourteen, almost a young woman, and I was startled as I realized the swiftness of the passage of time. She came to ask me to go and see her mother, and I went within the hour.

Busy as I was, I did not leave immediately after I had prescribed for her. A strange attraction held me by the fire. I observed that she still had no thought for herself, that her eyes constantly followed her daughter about the room. Everything was unchanged save that it was now the girl who watched by the bed. She followed me out of the house to hear what I thought of her mother's condition. Straight and brave she stood as I tried to prepare her for the inevitable.

Concern for the little girl and her unequal struggle continued in my thoughts as I drove about. I considered every possibility of helping her.

That afternoon I drove to the old Lindoll home where Maggie's sister, still unmarried, lived alone. The great house seemed to retire farther and farther up the path as I approached it. The blinds of many windows were closed. An old servant took my hat and coat and ushered me into the drawing room. Despite the grandeur of the room, it carried an air of stuffiness and a faint odor of mothballs amid its thick carpet and velvet hangings. From their cracked and faded frames old family portraits looked glumly out, some down at me and others haughtily the other way. The fine old furniture carried a feeling that it was rarely used. Several logs rested on the brass andirons, but there was no fire and no ashes of a former one.

Hearing a step behind me, I arose to meet Maggie's sister. She was dressed in black silk with a high collar edged in white and was more stooped and withered than I had remembered her. I briefly stated the object of my visit.

"No," she said firmly, "Maggie wouldn't listen to me and disgraced the family. She allowed her husband to call for a settlement at a time I could ill afford to make one. She has had her part. If she is in want, it is no affair of mine."

I told her of Maggie's life—of its courage, its nobility. I mentioned the little girl, the last member of her family. Nothing I could say would persuade her to change her position. Further talk was useless. I felt a sense of relief when I was out in the open air and the sunshine again.

It was a losing fight from the start. Maggie slowly became weaker. One day I sat by her bed and looked through the window. The ground was covered with snow.

"Yes, it is beautiful," said Maggie in answer to my comment, "and then it is a change; but I don't know that I think it more beautiful than it has been all winter with the earth brown and the pattern of the bare branches against the dim, purple mountains and the slate-colored sky. Look at that maple. It is like some giant crystal, and just beyond it is an ash with its straight limbs and regular pattern. That beech beside the stream and the sycamores are still different, and there is a silver birch with its delicate, plume-like branches. As pretty as it all is, it is no prettier than it was when the leaves were green with summer or when they took on their autumn coloring.

"Last fall I awoke in the middle of the night. The moon was full, and it was almost as light as day. Down the slope I could see mist tangled in all the yellow leaves of the orchard and so little Maggie and I dressed and walked through it. I love it all '. . . seedtime and harvest, and cold and heat, and summer and winter, and day and night . . .'[5] I have loved life in its pleasure and ease, and I have loved it in its sorrow and toil. God has been good. He has given it all to me and now that he is holding out his hand for mine, I appreciate all the more his greatest gift, an immortality that I can see and understand." She looked lovingly at her daughter.

"Of course, I know," she continued after a pause, "that little Maggie may not be as fortunate as I have been. She may never live to have a child, but I like to think that I have at least passed the torch to other hands."

A few weeks later she wrote to the sister, whom she had not seen for years. As I expected, the message went unanswered.

After that there was little apparent change until the spring morning when Maggie rapidly grew worse. She asked me to send for her sister and, upon my sending word that if she wished to see Maggie alive she must come at once, her car was driven to the door. Though her chauffeur stood and held the car door open for her, she sat a full minute with a my-what-have-they-come-to expression written upon her face. Coming in, she surveyed the bare hall. There was a movement as if to

---

5. Genesis 8:22 (King James Version).

lay her wrap down; but then, as if reluctant to allow it to touch the poor chair, she hesitated and with the garment upon her arm entered Maggie's room and closed the door. My mind now swept through all those years and had come down to the present.

Still, I sat in the hall, and still there was no sound from within the room. It couldn't be long. Again, I looked to the fire, then far out over the fields and on to the sunset. I thought of Maggie's awareness of the miracle of nature, of her thankfulness to God for the experience of life, of the joy she had in living it, and of the transcendent value she had placed upon her child—the child that would carry her own life into the future.

The door of Maggie's room was opened, and my name was called. One glance was enough. I saw Maggie lying white and still on the bed and the great mass of brown hair of another Maggie, kneeling beside her.

The sister followed me from the room. I stood and looked at her expensive dress and jewels.

"She wanted me to take the girl," she said.

"Are you going to do so?" I asked.

"I suppose it is my duty and I have never failed in that. My! How like her father she looks!"

"I think she is the living image of her mother," I replied.

"Then you don't remember him," she said. "Poor Maggie! What a wreck she made of her life! She had as much as I did— enough, if she had not married, to have kept her in comfort."

The Family History

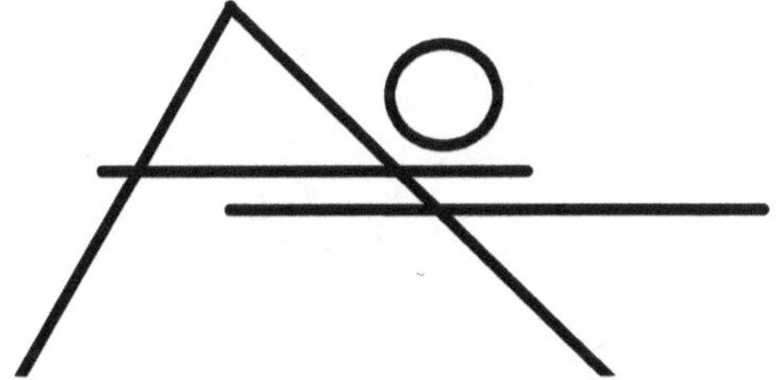

The Family History

There was something she wanted to say to me—something that was of importance to that pensive girl who followed me about the hall after telling me that she never knew her father, in fact, never had a father. A chance remark of mine was prompting her to speak. Then, by a twist of fate, the recollection of this same remark threw me into such confusion that I missed what she would have said. It may be as well, for the incident probably suggested to my mind a deeper meaning and made a more lasting impression than could have any actual words.

The untold part of a far nobler tale than this contains its very essence. The Master stooped down and with his finger wrote upon the sand. Were those marks a tabulation of crimes committed by those peering over his shoulder, were they an explanation of his intended course, or were they not, rather, marks traced in a moment of abstraction, unintelligible to those about him, yet representing all the conflicting thought, the emotions, and compassion with which this subject has been viewed through the ages? Were the actual words purposely not given to us so that each in accordance with his own light, in his own time, might interpret them in his own best way? Did not the very fact that the words were written on that shifting, changing medium—blurred by the first gust of wind, effaced by the tread of the first passerby—give to them their real permanence, make them more enduring than if written on parchment or engraved on stone, impress them upon the human heart forever?

It was the girl's last day in the hospital. It seemed almost impossible that she had entered it only a week before. Her illness had started as a little thing. Through neglect it had grown to alarming proportions by the time she entered the hospital. Upon her arrival I made a hasty examination and ordered her prepared for an emergency operation. She was just out of her teens, unmarried and girlish. Though tall, she seemed little more than a child. Her relatives were not present and she herself, having said she was of age, signed the permit for the operation.

After the operation I walked into the waiting room to talk to her family. They were not there. Thinking they would be by her bedside, I went to her ward.

"No," said the nurse, "there has been no one. Perhaps they will come soon."

The patient rallied quickly and through the next few days made a uniformly rapid improvement. Thus, there being no uneasiness on my part, there was no real reason to discuss her condition with her family, and so I made no further attempt to see them, though I remember that I did think it odd that I never chanced to meet them on my rounds.

There were no visitors, no flowers, no get-well cards of sympathy and love and encouragement such as litter the tables and are pinned to the curtains of so many of our sick rooms. She did not seem to miss them. She never complained. Though I never saw her smile and she spoke no more words than necessary, she was always agreeable and pleasant in a quiet, self-effacing way. Each day I visited her. Each day I noticed more and more the strange quietness of her manner and was more impressed by the simple, elemental viewpoint she held on every subject brought up.

Presently she was out of bed and about the ward. Her light wrap brought out all the more the frailty of her thin form—its tall and slender, yet childlike, lines. Soon now she was well enough to be discharged from the hospital.

That last day I took her chart from the rack at the hall desk and went into the ward. My patient was dressed and ready to leave. Together we entered the privacy and comfort of a small reception room. She listened attentively to my brief instructions, said that she would obey them, and then in her simple way thanked me for my care.

I took out my pen. "I noticed," I said to her, "that your family history is incomplete. Will you give it to me now? Is your father well?"

There was a slight hesitation and then, "I never knew my father," she said in a quiet, low voice.

"When did he die?" I asked.

"I never had a father," she replied.

This then was the reason for the omission. Her eyes were turned to mine. Then all at once I saw from what depths of her soul those words had come. In that moment I saw all the years of longing, of taunts, of insecurity, of sadness. I spoke a few kindly words that I do not remember. Then, thinking it might help, I attempted to change her wistfulness into resolution.

"It has a real meaning for you and will help in one way," I said. "You will see to it that when you have a little girl, she will have a father, won't you? Every child has a right to a father."

She made no reply, not the slightest movement, but by then I knew her well enough to know that it was a studied calm. At that moment I heard my name on the auto call and so did not finish her chart. Gathering it up, I told her good-bye and left the room.

At the door a nurse met me with a dressing cart. Together we went down the hall to see a patient in another room. On the way my mind was still with the girl, and I recalled how much a father could mean to and give to his daughter—his delight at her birth: the trips, first in his arms and then on his back; someone for the little girl to look to and love; the mainstay of the home; and, united in love with the mother, security, stability, and happiness.

Shortly after reaching the room, I was attracted by a soft footfall and glanced up in time to see the girl walk slowly past the door. As she did so, she dropped from my thoughts.

Concerned now about my new patient, my mind left the girl completely; so completely that it was not until later that I realized she had been standing by the door as I came from the room on my way to the nurses' desk, her chart still in my hand.

At the desk I wrote the discharge on the chart and had begun to give it a last-minute check-up for any missing details when I became aware of the slender form of the girl standing silently, close beside me. Still intent on my work, I felt subconsciously that in a moment I would be finished with the record and free to explain my instructions to her if that were what she wished.

Then, all at once I saw the fateful line, "She has one child, a girl, two years old." The admitting clerk had written it a week before. If I had read it at all, in the anxiety and haste of that day it had been forgotten. Then it would have made no impression upon me. Now it burned itself into my mind—as changeless as the fact that it records.

I glanced up. Her face was drawn and deathly pale as she looked down at the words.

In confusion and regret I realized what pain my remark must have caused. I arose, said some meaningless thing, and turned away. Not waiting for the elevator, I opened a nearby door leading to the stairs. I glanced back and saw her standing as I see her now, motionless, her eyes still staring at the open chart.

Time

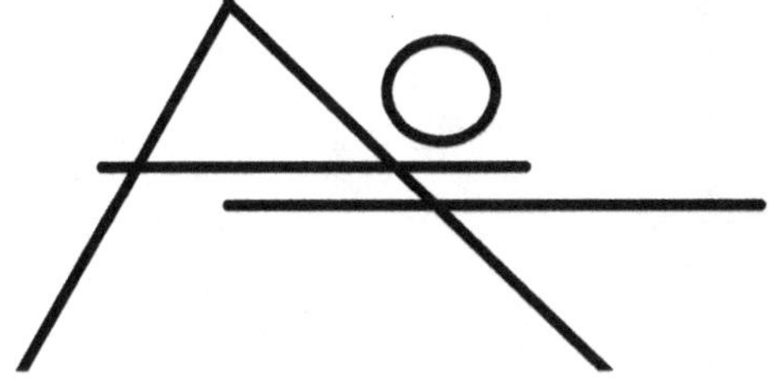

Time

It is impossible to step twice into the same river.

Heraclitus

It was as if some church had just let out and the members of the congregation were still loitering about. Men dressed in their best and women with their pretty gowns and bright-colored parasols were coming down the high, broad steps of the auditorium, standing in groups upon the lawn as they chatted with one another or strolling along the white colonnades. A general reunion of all the classes of the medical school was being held on the university campus that bright June day.

Since the days when I had been a student there, my own class had held many reunions. I had attended none of these. Even before I left school, the First World War had been declared. This meant for me a long term in the military forces—years of stress that made faint the memory of all that had gone before, that so nearly blotted from my mind the names and images of my classmates, that, try as I might, my roommate, and my roommate only, could I remember. It was several years after the war had ended before I was able to recall these lost images, dim they were at first, then clearer and clearer, yet never as they had been before. For, though I did not realize it then, those salvaged memories had acquired a new element—one of fixity—that in some way endowed my classmates with an attribute of eternal youth that we bestow upon those who died young and long ago.

Even as these returning memories awakened within me the desire to pay a visit to my old school, another factor came forward to cry for the visit's postponement. This factor was a large surgical practice that carried with it responsibilities not easy to leave. Now, after many years, these cares had been lifted somewhat and, responding to an invitation from the secretary of the Alumni Association, I had arrived with the anticipation of renewing the friendships of my college days and of walking again upon the campus of that magnificent and beautiful institution which, in memory, lay so close to my heart.

It was the old place and yet it was not. The growth the institution had made was remarkable. Building after building sprawled far beyond the original campus. The little cluster of old buildings that I had known now formed but the heart of a great modern university.

Despite the welcome and friendliness that everywhere prevailed, a sense of strangeness hung over the scene. The growth of the institution and the material changes did not entirely account for this feeling. It was something else. Though the campus lay fair before me and though I could give many details of my stay there, there was still an air of unreality about it—that strange quality which sometimes hangs over a new place giving one the feeling that though he cannot quite remember when, he has been there before, perhaps in some half-forgotten dream, perhaps in another life.

Earlier that day, at the office of the Alumni Association, I had been told that though several members of my class were expected, none had yet arrived. Surely by now they had come.

From group to group I wandered, looking for my friends. I exchanged a few light words with many whom I met, but for me there were no remembered faces. Several times I thought that I recognized someone, but when I stopped him, I found I was mistaken. Mistaken too were several other men who came forward to call me by a name other than my own. As this continued and I met no one whom I knew, to the sense of strangeness that I had felt at first was added the numbing chill of loneliness.

Here and there I walked alone, through the wisteria and boxwood gardens and among those stately buildings. The blue dome of the rotunda with its glittering stars now seemed far above me, farther than it had ever seemed before. I visited the war memorials and read the names of those who had given their lives in those titanic struggles. Many of these names I had known and loved—a number far greater than the number of those I would recognize upon the roster of the reunion. I read and pondered the beautiful inscriptions on the memorials. One quotation held an especial meaning for me that day. In Lawrence Binyon's poem, "For the Fallen", it says: "They shall grow not old, as we that are left grow old: / Age shall not weary them, nor the years condemn."[6]

As I walked upon the campus, I visited the bronze statues of the illustrious men who had been associated with the university. How real these men had seemed to me as a student, how close to me they had been, how I had looked to them for

---

6. Lawrence Binyon, "For the Fallen," *Oxford Book of English Verse*, ed. Arthur Quiller-Couch (New York: Oxford University Press, 1941), 1090, lines 13-14.

inspiration and had found it! Now it was with a sense of failure and futility that I stood before their statues. These statesmen and leaders of men now seemed foreign and far away.

How had they looked at their own lives? I wondered. They had reached the pinnacle, the very zenith of life's accomplishments and achievements, but was even that enough? Was it possible that they too had felt when their labors were over that they had accomplished little?

A few of the classrooms and laboratories were open, deserted, and lonely. Most of them were closed and locked against me. Once they had been mine, but now there was no sense of possession, of their belonging to me or I to them. I was a stranger on what had once been my own doorstep.

The university, having nurtured us in her womb, had labored and brought us forth, I thought as the alumni streamed about me. Others will come forth, but for us there is no return.

The officers of the association were doing everything possible to entertain the alumni. Tours of the new buildings were being conducted, lectures given, and clinics were being held at the amphitheater. These were not for one in my mood.

At the hospital I made inquiry about my old professors. None were on the staff. The young woman at the information booth had never heard of most of them.

Thinking that I would rest a little before crossing the campus to see my old room on the Range, I took a seat in the lobby. Presently some young men began to stroll in, one or two at a time, for their mail. They were hardly more than boys. Their faces were fresh with the bloom of youth still upon their cheeks; their eyes and teeth, shining. Their hair was short cut, clean, fresh, and lustrous. They wore white coats and carried stethoscopes in their pockets. They stopped at the counter, leaned upon it with their elbows, and talked and flirted a little with the pretty girls working there.

Who are they? I wondered. Then the truth slowly came to me. They were the interns. Once I had been one of them.

A member of the welcoming committee came into the lobby and seeing me sitting alone he came over. I told him my name and class. He gave me the name of a classmate who had come.

"He is in the hospital now," he said. "You have only to wait here to see him. More will come."

I scrutinized every person who came through. I had almost given up hope when a tired-looking man of advanced age came from the hall. There was a faint response from within and, summoning my courage, I went to him and called him by name. It was he. I had thought of him the day before, but then he lived in his youth. It was if he had aged and withered in a single night.

We exchanged greetings. He spoke of the absent members, how few were left. Then upon questioning we told briefly of our families and our work. I sensed at once that we had nothing in common save the fact that we had once been there together.

He had an appointment and said, "good-bye." He bore the name of one of my classmates, yet strange he seemed, and different.

As I crossed the campus again, visions, first of these, as I had remembered them, and then of others, kept coming to my mind. Upon the Range I attempted to identify that particular green shutter which guarded the heavy wooden door of the little room where I had lived. I thought I knew the number, but when I came to the one I had in mind, I was not sure. My roommate could have told me. He had kept up with the happenings of the university, had attended many of the smaller reunions and had many times written to tell me any news of importance; but I had not heard from him now in several years. He was not here. He had not come.

In our school days he had a beautiful singing voice and sang in the church choir and the glee club. In fancy I could hear him now, somewhat vaguely, singing as he came across the campus. Try as I might, I could not quite make out the words.

Increasingly now, friends and activities of the old days came into view. From where I stood, in memory I could look under the Range into the large room where the Saturday night parties had been held.

The throng of men and women of the reunion flowed about me. They were felt more than seen, as were the new buildings. They slowly vanished from my consciousness, and I wandered in a vague land, upon some mystic campus, some Germelshausen[7] risen for a day. Through it I walked, lost in thought and memory, seeing naught but those vague half-remembered forms of the past. As I walked along the arched promenade of the Range, I looked through the heavy closed doors as if they were non-existent, and into the rooms where sat at their desks the vaporous forms of my old friends. Upon every

---

7. Friedrich Gerstacker, *Germelshausen*, trans. Isaac Bachman (PA: Handy Book, 1916). Germelshausen is the enchanted German village that rises from the marsh for one day every hundred years.

path some beloved professor, now long since engulfed by time, lifted his hat in return of my salute. It was a land of memories, a shadowy land peopled with ghosts of the past.

I was awakened from my trance-like dream by the consciousness of men hurrying across the campus and converging to a flight of steps that led downhill to the hospital.

"What is going on?" I asked a man as he passed.

"Dr. Rankin is here," he replied. "Some of the fellows have been after him to give his old lecture on senile insanity. The scheduled speaker has offered to stand aside for him, and Dr. Rankin has consented to deliver the lecture."

My heart leaped. Here was something that struck a responsive chord. Dr. Rankin had been our professor of mental diseases. His lecture on senile insanity had been the highlight of the course. It was the lecture for which he was noted. I too would again hear this wonderful lecture and, when that was over, I would—I would shake his hand and talk of old times and find myself again. I joined the crowd and hurried toward the amphitheater.

Once again, as in my student days, I sat in the great oval room with its tier after tier of seats, now filled with strangers, and gazed down upon the stage. There I had seen wonderful, kindly surgeons operate. There I myself had lent them my amateurish assistance. There, now, in less than half an hour would be re-enacted a scene I had thought of many times in the years that had passed. The principal actor would be a man marvelous in intellect and power.

As I sat and waited, my mind carried me back through all those years. In memory I was a student again and in that memory an old man sat upon this same stage and Dr. Rankin, strong and youthful, stood beside him.

"Thank you for coming. Please tell me your name," Dr. Rankin requested kindly.

The old man gave his name.

"Your age?"

"I do not know."

"Do you remember your mother and her name?"

"Oh yes." The old man's impassive face lit up.

"Your father?"

"Yes."

"How many brothers and sisters did you have? Can you give their names?"

"I had three brothers and one sister." He gave their names.

"Where did you go to school?"

Now the old man began to falter. Finally, he named an elementary school.

"Were you married?"

"Yes," answered the old man after some thought.

"What was your wife's name?"

"Mary," he finally said as he groped back through the years.

"Mary what? What was her maiden name?"

"I have forgotten," the old man said at last.

"Did you have any children?"

"Yes, I think so . . . I don't know. I am not sure," he faltered.

"What became of your wife? Do you know?"

"No."

"When did you come here?"

"I don't know," he said with a slight shake of the head.

"Do you know what day it is, what year?"

Each of these last questions was answered with a shake of the head.

"Have you had lunch today?" There was no reply.

"Let me show your keys to the class," Dr. Rankin said gently and having put his fingers into the old man's vest pocket, he let drop a gold chain from which hung a Phi Beta Kappa and other keys. The professor evidently had secreted them there for effect.

"This man," he said, turning to us, "was a scholar. Long before I knew him personally, I knew of the honors he had won at the university. He became one of the ablest lawyers in the state.

"In infancy and childhood," Dr. Rankin then told us, "the mind is fresh and impressionable. Each imprint upon it leaves a memory deep and sharp. Time passes. Each new impression is now superimposed upon former ones. As countless millions are recorded and the tissues themselves become older and older, the impressions ever tend to become more shallow and less vivid. Throughout life this process progresses until finally such impressions as are made are superficial and transitory.

"These last impressions are the ones that disappear first when the blood vessels to the brain begin to harden and nutrition to that all-important organ begins to be reduced. The process now reverses itself. One by one the lighter, more recent impressions are erased until there is left but a great, blank gap of empty years between an old man's present moment and his past—a past which moves with his ever-receding memory. As each day's remembrances in their turn grow dim, the next ones, having nothing overlaying them, become clearer and brighter until they also fade, to be replaced by others still further back."

Step by step Dr. Rankin retraced the path the old man had trod. He spoke of the old man's boyhood, of the brooks and the fields, of his first gun, his dog.

"Slowly, relentlessly, the degeneration increases," Dr. Rankin continued. "Himself a child again, the old man lives among children and their toys. They are those of the long ago. For him the hearth fire burns again. Back, back is carried the threshold of his memory until that last vision, the image of his mother, fades and, within that mind, desolation lies where once warm memories and love and reason dwelt.

"When I look at you fine young men," Dr. Rankin said, slowly turning his eyes from one of us to another, "it is hard for me to realize that every one of you who will live long enough will come to this."

Dr. Rankin's words spoken so many years ago still carried their dread prophecy.

How much of it? I wondered, could he repeat?

The amphitheater door opened. A feeble old man leaning heavily on his cane slowly advanced. His clothes hung loosely upon him as if he had rapidly lost weight.

It is the patient, I thought.

The spectators, a few at first, one here and one there, stood; and then the others, hesitatingly, as if not quite sure of the reason for doing so, also arose.

"It is Dr. Rankin," someone whispered. My heart sank.

All remained standing until the old professor had advanced into the circle, had acknowledged the salute, and had waved his hand for them to be seated.

I should not have expected time to withhold its hand from him while it changed all else, I thought.

Now came an intern carrying a small straight chair and leading another old man. He placed the chair in the center of the stage and in it seated the patient.

Dr. Rankin spoke a few words of welcome to the audience, gave a brief introduction, and then turned to the old man in the chair.

"What is your name?" he asked.

The patient answered the question.

"How old are you?"

After a pause came the answer, "I do not know."

"What is your trouble?"

"I have no trouble. I am very comfortable."

Dr. Rankin stared at him as if puzzled by the answer. He then turned and again looked upward to the throng in the amphitheater. As one lost in a maze, he scanned the faces before him. At length his eyes rested upon a man he recognized. It was his friend, the Dean.

"Why are we here?" he asked, bewildered.

An absolute silence fell upon the room. Every eye was fixed upon the face of the old master.

In that atmosphere of suspended animation, that rapt and silent group, the old professor's image was thrown into high relief.

"Don't you remember?" replied the Dean. "You came to give your lecture on senile insanity."

"I did? Why was I going to do that?" asked Dr. Rankin.

Now the Dean was at his side.

"I am afraid you shouldn't have come today," he said. "It is very warm. Let us go now. We will call on you at another time if we may."

They slowly led him out. The door closed behind him. Still, with all the rest, I stood in silence. Quietly then I stole from the room, made my way to my car, to my place in the present—and with that ever-flowing moment moved on.

Permanent Disability

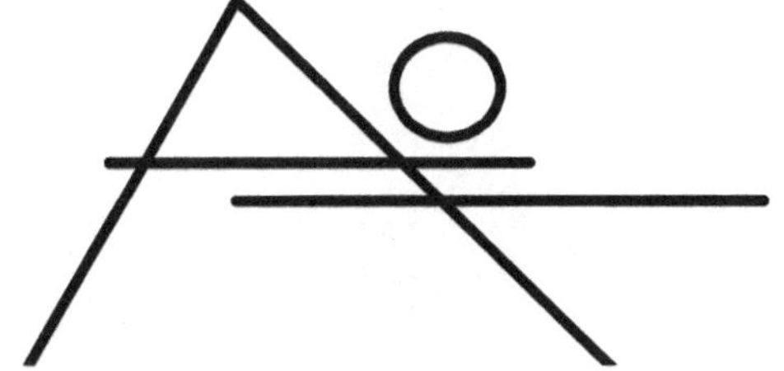

Permanent Disability

In the morning mail I received the following letter. It was partly a form letter, partly made up of interpolations.

Mr. George Platte
Pinola Rd.
Rt. #2

In re: Claim no. 253-337 L

Dear Doctor:

The claimant designated above is insured under one of our group policies. At your earliest convenience, please visit the claimant at his home and make a medical examination in connection with his claim under this insurance policy. After a careful physical examination please give us your diagnosis, prognosis, and if the claimant is disabled an estimate of future disability. We are essentially interested in your opinion, not the opinion of the claimant. As the claim is based on a throat condition, you are hereby authorized to take with you a specialist of your own selection to assist in this part of the examination.

Enclosed is a form that we use in connection with disability claims and upon which we would like to have you make your report. Please send your report, along with the bill for your services, to the medical division.

If for any reason you cannot conduct the examination, please notify the writer of this letter to that effect.

Thank you for your cooperation.

Upon inquiry, I found that Pinola was a dirt road turning off the black top in the Luther Section, several miles from the city.

Why not? I thought. I was not expected to treat him, some other doctor was doing that. All the insurance company wanted me to do was to see whether he was still disabled. There was evidently no hurry. I could choose my own time and my own company. A trip in the country with my good friend, Dr. Ted Goodruff, the specialist I should ask to accompany me, would be a pleasant way to spend an hour or two.

"Sure! Would love to go; but I can't go today, old fellow," said Ted over the telephone when I called him. "In a day or two—why not let me call you, and we will try to get together."

It was several days before Dr. Goodruff telephoned to say that he could get off to make the trip. This time it was I who could not leave my work.

"I am snowed under," I explained. "Let's make it the last of the week. How would Saturday just after lunch do? Do you mind working Saturday afternoon?"

"Not a bit! I will come by for you Saturday, sure. Go with me in my new car. I want to show it to you."

On Saturday he called. "Well, it looks like we are going to have to put it off again," he sang out in his cheery voice. "It rained all night. I wouldn't like to get stuck in the mud, you know." And he laughed merrily.

"All right, the first of the week," I said. "Be certain to call me."

In the press of work the request of the insurance company completely dropped from my mind. A week later my secretary asked me a question about an insurance form. This reminded me of my neglected duty and I called Dr. Goodruff at once.

"Let's go now," I insisted. "It has been two weeks. The company will be writing to me again the first thing we know."

"How about tomorrow at two o'clock?" he asked. "If that is all right, I'll come for you rain or shine."

It was a clear, fine day for the trip, somewhat crisp and windy but the earth was dry. I had asked my operating room supervisor to put into a package everything she thought might be needed, and with this surprisingly large bundle under my arm, I waited at the hospital door until Dr. Goodruff drove up. He also was well equipped with a very large bag and a small one.

As we leisurely drove along, Ted made the journey a merry one by drawing from his wonderful fund of amusing stories and remembrances. We inquired our way a time or two. At length, we came to a very poor and unattractive section and finally drove up a steep hill. At its very crest stood a country store which evidently was the one that had been cited as our landmark, for it answered the description of an old, worn-out building covered with red imitation-brick tar paper now hanging in tatters.

I went into the store for further directions. Yes, I learned, Pinola Road turned off here—in fact, right against this store. Mr. Platte lived in one of a row of small houses about a mile down the road. No, there wouldn't be any number and the storekeeper could not say in just which house he lived, but suggested that we inquire again when we reached the houses.

Slowly we drove along, talking. Presently we sighted the houses, six or eight unpainted shacks close together, to the right of and near the road. They were the only signs of human habitation in all that barren waste.

At the same time, we saw something else that held our attention. In front of one of these houses was a funeral party, made up of a small group of people, three or four old cars, a hearse with open doors, and pallbearers who were now carrying a black casket down the walk.

Dr. Goodruff pulled his car off the road and stopped. We watched the casket being put into the hearse and saw the doors close. All present save one woman climbed into the cars and the procession slowly filed past us. The lone woman turned and entered the house.

"Platte must live in one of these houses," I said. "Let's ask her which one."

Getting out, I took my bundle and Ted his bags. We walked up the steps to the rickety porch and knocked on the still-open door. The woman—rawboned, graying, with an expressionless face—came to the door.

"Will you please tell us where Mr. Platte lives?" I asked.

"What do you want with him?" she demanded suspiciously.

"We want to examine him for the insurance company," I replied.

She stood on the high step of the doorway and looked down at us for what seemed to be a full minute. Then she crossed the porch and walked out upon the yard. We followed. She stooped low, one hand on her knee, looked and then pointed down the road in the direction the procession had taken.

"Well, all I can say," she drawled, "is that if you are going to examine him you'd better hurry."

A Stranger Here

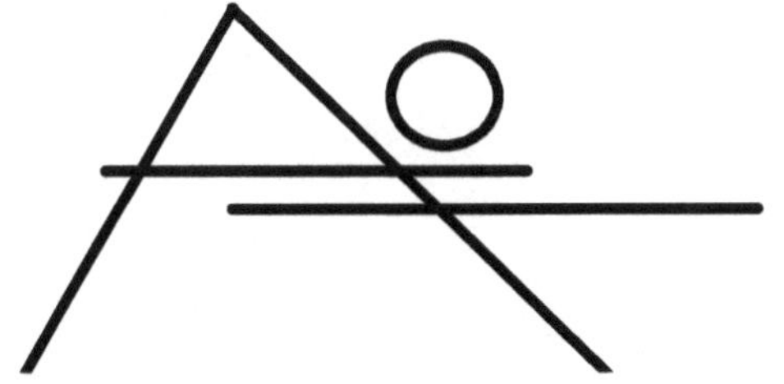

A Stranger Here

That black night of eternity, that vast space in which the past, the present and the future are one, is not a silent void. It is a night filled with strange, vast dreams. For a Spirit dwells therein that everywhere moves, that from the very stress of the vacuum has created energy, and that from this energy has collected the enormous mass of the whirling, flaming stars that in those stupendous reaches are but cold points of light set in eternal darkness. Around these stars it has spun other bodies on which are illimitable oceans and mountains of stone and has planted upon these—strangest of all the wonders that have been drawn from that limitless well—the miraculous process we call life.

It is with this last, precious, vaporous entity that the doctor is concerned—its preservation, its development, and its happiness. Life in all its varied and changing forms is his interest. He is awed by its coming and its departure, moved by its emotions, delighted by its physical and intellectual achievements, rapt and lost in thought and meditation as he contemplates its source and its relations to its environment.

Are life and breath and spirit synonymous in fact as well as in word or is the last something else? Did life upon this earth develop here, spontaneously, within an arrangement and rearrangement of atoms and molecules; or had an essence, a leaven, been brought in by a meteorite from the boundless depths of space? Who can tell? We know only that the process was established early in some warm marsh near the sea. It was there that life, having no substance itself, existed and acted within substance. Gradually it extended, selecting, but still limited to the substances within reach, it ever increased this reach and built from its surroundings a greater and a more suitable habitat for itself. The water of the ocean was used, its suspended salts, the earth, the air, the sunshine. Ever renewing itself, ever reaching out, ever developing, it built into its habitat the sky and the sunset until at last a form of beauty, intelligent and ingenious beyond belief, capable of surpassing nobility, emerged—man—man with his ability to think, to contemplate this process, to feel that this marvelous entity of life is a part of the eternal, and at last to call his own body the temple of the Spirit.

Withal, the body of man is still tied into its surroundings as surely as the tree which presses its mouth to the earth. The body of man, formed from the elements of its early environment, upon these same elements depends every day, every moment for its replenishment, its restoration, its survival, and at last returns these same elements to the great fund.

Between his coming and his departure each man adds some small amount of original thought, of combination, of invention to the sum total of human knowledge. Slowly, gradually, from countless hands and minds through the ages, the civilization we know today has developed. A child and then a man, growing into this civilization, does not at once realize that it is not the normal—does not realize that our now vast sum of knowledge, our machines, clothes, customs, literature, and music are but a slowly and a painfully accumulated superstructure in which we move as if it were reality.

Man occasionally, when time affords or when moved by some strange happening, gazes to the heavens and heavenly bodies as he would to some dim and unknown shore. To his mind may come a fleeting question of the secret which it holds, a fleeting question as to his own place within its vastness, perchance a moment of vague longing.

Under the great lights of the operating room one night such a moment came to me.

As oft repeated as the scene may be, for me that night it created a profound emotion and a lasting memory—a memory of a strange, unearthly visitation, when the veil that separates the ephemeral from the permanent was for a moment drawn aside and I saw our world as through the eyes of one from the realms of the absolute.

Earlier that night, having made a professional call in the country, I was being driven toward the city by the father of the patient I had just left. The car was warm and comfortable. The radio was on and, as we sped along the great superhighway, I listened to the wild beat of its music and to the news from a battlefield halfway around the world.

Although at that time I was hardly conscious of the sights along the way, they recurred to me with startling vividness a little later. The highway was filled with cars and great trucks rolling with their freight. In them rode men, eager, driven onward by urgency and the fierce competition of life. There was the blast of a locomotive horn, its headlight's glare, and then came the rush of the speeding train with flash after flash of light as it hurtled past. The lights of the city came into view along with the factories with their glow on the sky and the great freight yards, alive with action, as the provisions to sustain the city another day were unloaded.

Having arrived at the terminal, I bade good-bye to my driver, left his car for an electric train, and was soon crossing the river on a great bridge swung by its cobweb of steel. A fleet of battleships with its carriers was standing down the river. Its signals were flashing back and forth. The lights along the shore converged across the water to me in shining, rippling paths. In the sky were the blinking and the roar of airplanes bound for all the ports of the earth. Millions of lights of the city shone in the windows of its lofty buildings.

The train, which had been gliding over the firm roadbed of the bridge, now quickened its speed. We descended rapidly and, with a violent swaying of the cars and an almost deafening roar, rushed underground. On we swept past the smaller stations, on through the black tube. In a matter of minutes, we arrived at my destination. I climbed the stairs and came out upon the street.

Brilliantly lighted and colored by electric signs, the street was thronged with people. Many more poured from the theaters. Some strolled along, some stopped to look into the display windows with their various devices and apparel. I passed the opera house. Men in tall hats and evening clothes and women bedecked in jewels and furs were being handed into their limousines by liveried footmen; others stood in groups chatting, blocking the sidewalk, unmindful of passersby, forced to walk around them, oblivious of hostile glances—some of envy, some of hatred. Still other people hastened onto the scene, and still others hastened away.

I took a cab and went to the hospital. An emergency had just been admitted.

The patient was a young woman, a prospective mother long overdue. She was almost exsanguinated, now kept alive by transfusions. It was flesh and blood once more, with all its fundamental weaknesses and kinship to death.

Though I was weary, still somewhat dazed, and perhaps not quite oriented after my long ride, the operation was quickly over and the patient returned to her room but without her baby. Its spark of life had returned to that eternal night from whence it came.

It was beautiful baby. That certain almost translucency of its skin made it seem as if evolution had reached its goal: a human being suitable to live an almost ethereal existence.

The noises of the street broke in—that of a bus as it increased its speed, the roar of a giant motor, and the sound of heavy pounding wheels.

I vaguely felt that the baby, that crowning product of all the ages, was too simple, too elemental, too closely related to the great forces of nature to have fitted the mold into which it would have been forced—that we had missed the way.

I stood beside the still form and gazed out upon man's struggle upward toward the light—his achievements since first he came to this world, as naked and as empty handed as this babe. I gazed upon those kaleidoscopic images that man has fashioned—apparently fixed for a moment but, by some strange parallax, in truth moving, shifting, changing, increasing, diminishing, and then, together with their maker, being swept away. I looked and marveled at their scope. Yet at no place, measured against the absolute, did it present completeness. There was no resting place. There was no hope for that phantom of peace that, like the dazzling promise at the rainbow's end, forever eludes man's search.

All at once life seemed indeed a fitful fever. Against the backdrop of that majestic calm where I stood, the world before me filled with turbulence and strife, and I, a wayfarer in a strange and alien land, with a tenure of a day. My real home seemed amid the stardust, beside the Mystic River.

Appendix

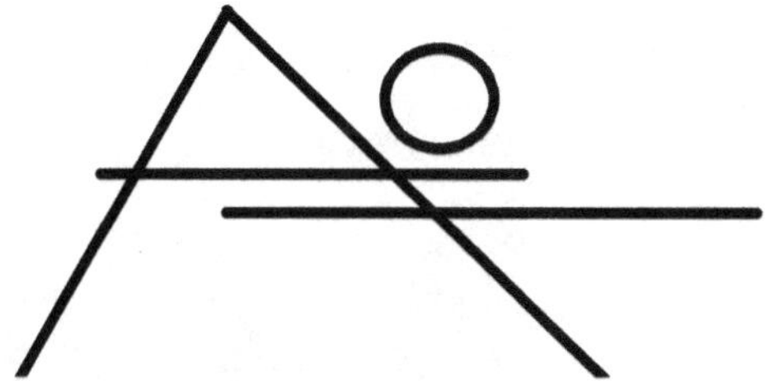

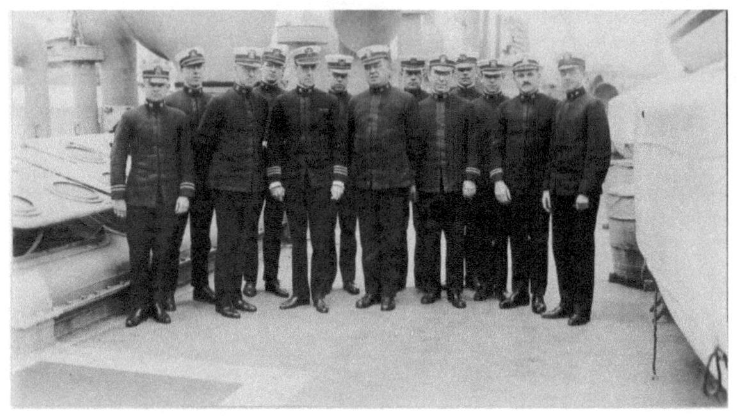

Officers of US hospital ship Comfort

April 6, 1919 Medical officer Lieutenant Charles S Norburn

front row far left[8]

---

8. War Department. 1789-9/18/1947s, accessed August 16, 2022, https:/
/catalog.archives.gov/id/4551109

Charles Strickland Norburn
1890-1990

1915

Graduated from University of North Carolina at Chapel Hill in Medical Program

1917

Graduated from Medical School at University of Virginia

Enlisted and accepted in the US Navy by an Act of Congress, graduating early due to his passing the physical and mental exams so brilliantly despite a physical deficiency (height)

1918

Served on the USS Havana and then USS Comfort for the duration of the war

1919

Rank Lieutenant (Jg), transferred to USS Comfort where his surgery first attracted particular attention

Promoted to Lieutenant

Transferred to Naval Hospital League Island, PA, Medical School

Awarded special course at Mayo Clinic at Mayo Clinic, Rochester, MN, being one of the first two men ever chosen for this course by the government

1920

Rank Lieutenant, Instructor of X-Ray at Naval Hospital
League Island, PA

1922

Transferred to Naval Hospital, Washington, DC

Visiting surgeon at Mayo Clinic, Rochester, MN

1923

Served on USS Mercy and USS Relief transporting American
Expedition Forces back from war—made several trans-Atlantic
trips

Selected by the US Surgeon General to accompany President
Warren Harding as his personal surgeon

Retired from the US Navy; lived and worked in Philadelphia
Moved back to Asheville, NC

1928

Worked in Asheville, NC and founded The Norburn Hospital
& Clinic on Montford Avenue with his brother

1929

Elected Fellow in American College of Surgeons

1930s-1940s

While growing his successful hospital and practice,
he marries Helen Johnson and begins raising a family

1946

Moved The Norburn Hospital & Clinic to Biltmore Avenue, Asheville, NC, greatly enlarging the hospital

1950

Sold The Norburn Hospital & Clinic to Victoria Hospital which then merged with other small hospitals to form Memorial Mission Hospital utilized his state of the art equipment and outstanding medical library, now a part of the MAHEC Health Science Library

Went into private practice in Biltmore, NC

Epilogue

A Rennaissance man, he had many interests and talents throughout his life

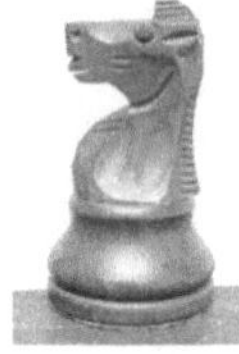

Enjoyed expert chess skills

Collected art and antiques

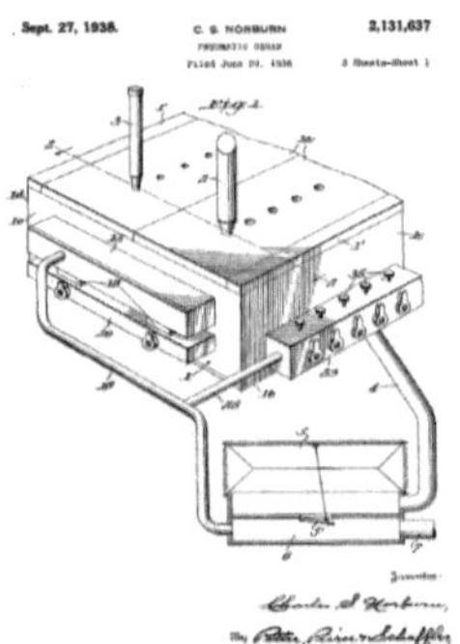

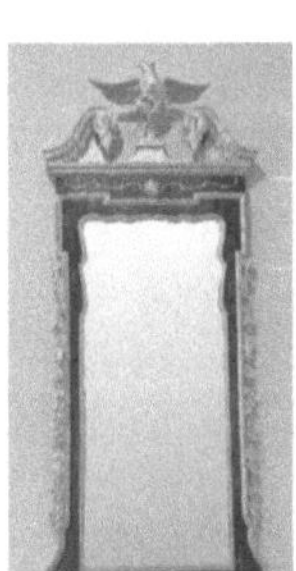

Designed and made fine wood furnishings in his home woodworking studio

Owned 3 pipe organs and obtained four patents for organ stops of his own design (technique is still used today)

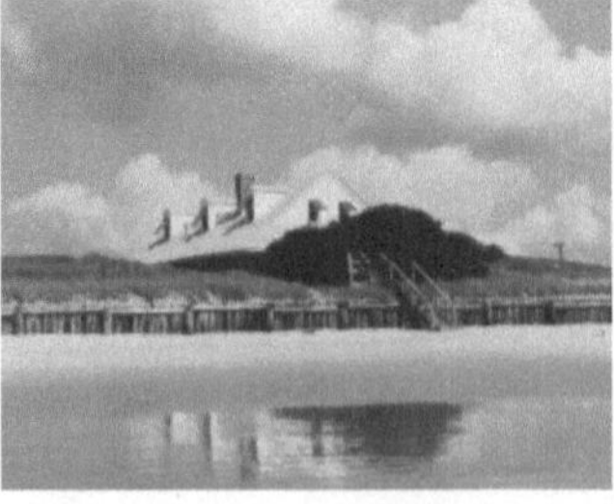

Restored the 18th century Nesbit/Norburn Beach house on Pawleys Island, SC for family summers and personal respite

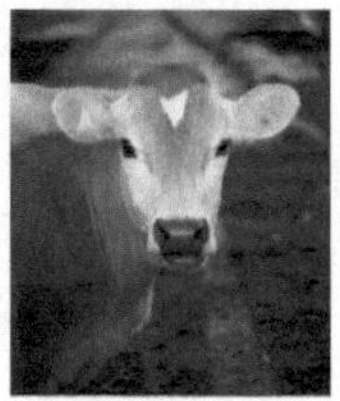

Had a small Guernsey dairy farm[9]

Author and published three books on the American monetary system in his 80s and 90s (the first book co-authored with his brother)

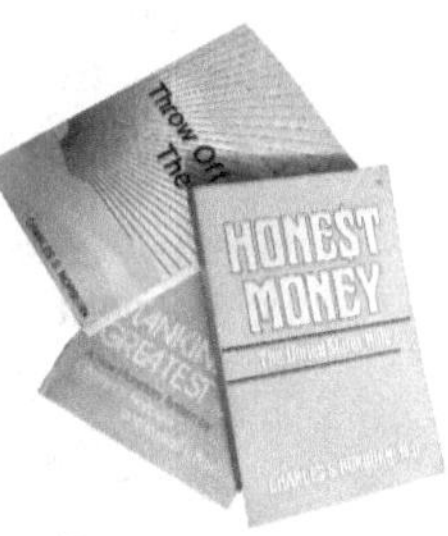

---

9. Jeremy Bishop, "Calf"," Photograph, accessed on August 12, 2022, https://www.unsplash.com

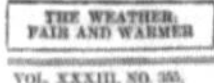

THE SUNDAY CITIZEN

THE WEATHER FAIR AND WARMER | 28 Pages Today
VOL. XXXIII, NO. 315. ASHEVILLE, N. C., SUNDAY MORNING OCTOBER 14, 1917. PRICE FIVE CENTS

THE SUNDAY CITIZEN, ASHEVILLE, N. C., OCTOBER 14, 1917.

DR. CHAS. S. NORBURN,
Former Asheville Boy With Atlantic Squadron.

An interesting war-time letter has been received from a former Asheville boy. Dr. Charles S. Norburn, whose achievements in order to serve his country have been of a rather remarkable nature. Dr. Norburn is now surgeon on the flag ship of the Atlantic squadron and from this responsible post writes letters glowing with enthusiasm concerning the privilege he feels the service of his country to be and giving such details of his surroundings and occupation as are permitted by the existing censorship. In order to demonstrate his patriotism by service Dr. Norburn applied for a position in the navy and while yet a student at the University of Virginia was, owing to his merit in scholarship, graduated ahead of time with the degree of doctor of medicine. In offering his services to the navy he relinquished an appointment as instructor in the University of Wisconsin, which position was to be assumed following his graduation from the University of Virginia. He then took the physical and mental examinations for the United States Navy and passing so brilliantly in the mental was accepted in view of this especial merit despite certain physical deficiencies [height]. Following hospital work in Philadelphia for the navy Dr. Norburn was ordered aboard the flag ship of the Atlantic fleet whose whereabouts is of course unknown. Dr. Norburn is also a graduate of the University of North Carolina. The following extracts from a

320

recent letter from this Asheville boy will interest many who know him and also those interested in details of existing conditions:

"The First Battalion of Marines left and took three of the doctors, so till others came in I had strenuous duties. Was on as officer of the day for forty hours at a stretch, night and day. Slept in a little room next to the office, but was up and down until I didn't do much of it. The job was not so much medicine as official, signing papers, detailing men, etc. Thought I would get off at noon at the end of the forty hours and rest a while. When I was handed orders to report immediately to the bureau of navigation. And as I was going, given verbal orders to take four hospital corpsmen to help deliver an insane patient to the naval hospital at Washington. Well, I did, and it caused me to miss by sleeper and so I waited until 10:30 p.m. and took a day coach and didn't sleep a bit. But I am right here and it is wonderful. A beautiful great battleship, not as large as the super-dreadnoughts, but which goes with and will fight with them. Unless you have been on one of this size you have no idea, just can't conceive how immense and substantial looking it all is. Just a floating world boiled down to the essentials and housed in steel. You can very easily get lost, I often do, but keep on going until I come to some landmark. Instead of the tent, here is my nice little room, about 7 X 15. Walls, roof and deck made from plate steel, painted light green. The deck (floor) is steel, of course, covered with dull brownish red, composition linoleum, painted on. The door is a sliding one, like a railwaydoor, but I never shut it. Its place is taken by heavy dark green draperies. Beautiful. Solid in color. The same hangings are about a little nook in which coats are kept, and also at the side of the head of my bed where I keep bath robe and slippers. The furniture looks like a Pullman car furniture, dark, heavy quartered oak matching the floor.

Bunk across the end, built in. Slide under it for shoes Dandy nice desk, very heavy, drawers reflected light, and covered with green felt. Pigeon-holes, etc. On the other side is a lavatory. Oak slab four feet wide against wall with nickel plated fixtures projecting; ten different ones. Wash basin folding up into it. Above this is case with mirrored front. There are five lights in the room. I keep them burning all day, for of course none of the cabins have port holes and is dark as pitch without them. Can turn them all off with one push of the button after I am in bed. Also I have a button which summons my boy. There is a blower about 8 inches in diameter which blows fresh air in all the time, also an electric fan at the head of my bed which I run most of the time. At night the boy asks what time I wish to be called, lays out my pajamas, calls me in the morning at 7:30, say, asks what I will have for breakfast, and departs. I proceed to a wonderful shower. No more cold Potomac for me at five a.m. Then descend into the ward room where my breakfast is ready by this time, and served. The breakfast consists of a choice of four or five fruits, any cereal, eggs anyway, etc., etc. The ward room is about seventy feet long, fixed up nicely with piano, pictures, trophies, books, etc., and some tables at one end. Two other large tables with green covers and heavy curved back leather chairs about them. At meal time, these are drawn out and put together in a long table with the chairs down the sides. About eighteen officers eat there, and the table is waited on by nine Philippinos. We get splendid fare; several courses even for lunch; baked squab, grape fruit already cut out to facilitate handling, and a band the "breathes fitfully music of the spheres" all day. Some of the men play chess, all play cards, bridge, cribbage, etc. The officers are very nice, and I like my superior medical officer a great deal.

Appendix

The "sick boy" is a dandy: isolation ward, dispensary ward, etc. Then there is a very nice operating room which they have just moved into a room behind armor. Of course, the other rooms and the ones we live in are not. There is not much doing in the sick line. When in port, there is an inspection of food coming aboard. At sea, there is not much doing. There are about a dozen patients. Sick call at 8:30 a.m. and 7:00 p.m. The doctors have to lecture once in two weeks to hospital men, and instruct them the band in little drills, but it is being said now that the last are useless, for in battle every water tight door will be closed and there will be no going down or aloft. Nothing will work but the guns. And we will be down in the third deck with a dozen water-tight great steel doors closed between us and the main deck. Even the ventilators are stopped. So I am afraid I wouldn't see much, even if we do get within range, unless I am detailed to a dressing station on the deck.

The guns are wonderful and the doctors are not considered non-combatants, either, as we are issued a 45 Colt automatic, which we keep as long as we are assigned to the ship."

Transcribed as printed from collection of Lillian N Alexander

Mayo Clinic

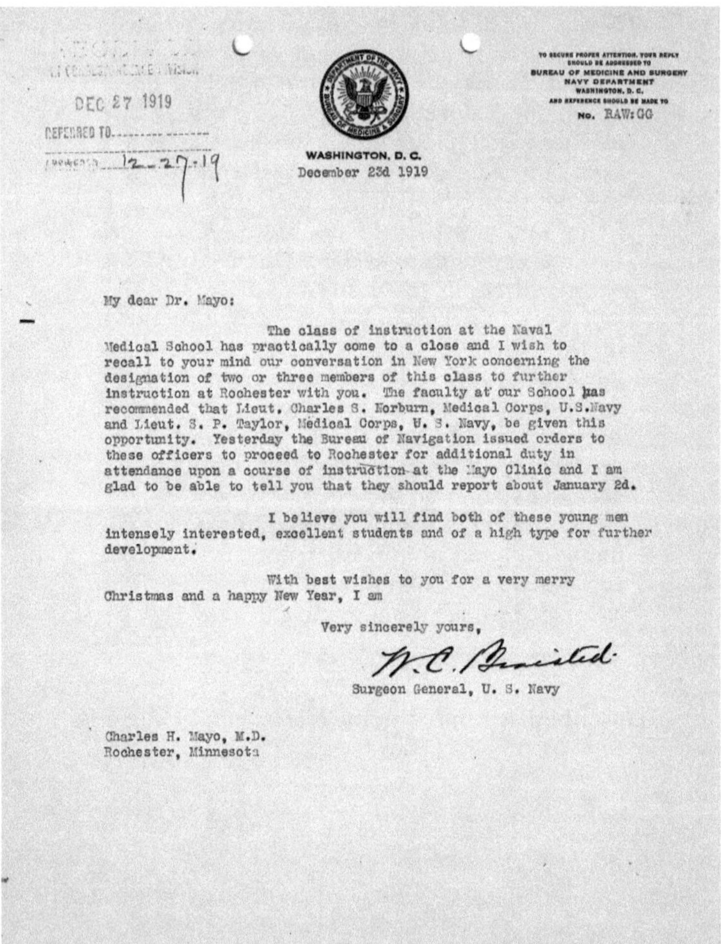

TO SECURE PROPER ATTENTION, YOUR REPLY
SHOULD BE ADDRESSED TO
BUREAU OF MEDICINE AND SURGERY
NAVY DEPARTMENT
WASHINGTON, D. C.
AND REFERENCE SHOULD BE MADE TO
No. RAW:GG

WASHINGTON, D. C.
December 23d 1919

DEC 27 1919

REFERRED TO..........

12-27-19

My dear Dr. Mayo:

The class of instruction at the Naval Medical School has practically come to a close and I wish to recall to your mind our conversation in New York concerning the designation of two or three members of this class to further instruction at Rochester with you. The faculty at our School has recommended that Lieut. Charles S. Norburn, Medical Corps, U.S.Navy and Lieut. S. P. Taylor, Medical Corps, U. S. Navy, be given this opportunity. Yesterday the Bureau of Navigation issued orders to these officers to proceed to Rochester for additional duty in attendance upon a course of instruction at the Mayo Clinic and I am glad to be able to tell you that they should report about January 2d.

I believe you will find both of these young men intensely interested, excellent students and of a high type for further development.

With best wishes to you for a very merry Christmas and a happy New Year, I am

Very sincerely yours,

W. C. Braisted

Surgeon General, U. S. Navy

Charles H. Mayo, M.D.
Rochester, Minnesota

Appendix

No. ....   N. M. S.

U. S. NAVAL MEDICAL SCHOOL

FOOT OF TWENTY-FOURTH STREET NW.

WASHINGTON, D. C.

December 30, 1919.

Doctor Charles H. Mayo,
     Rochester, N.Y.

My dear Doctor Mayo:

     This letter will introduce to you Doctors C.S.
Norburn and S. P. Taylor, of the Naval Medical Corps.
These officers are the ones Admiral Braisted wrote
you about a few days ago.

     Please allow me to express to you my great ap-
preciation of your kindness in offering the Surgeon
General and the Naval Medical Corps this opportunity
for post graduate work in surgery. I am sure that
Lieutenants Norburn and Taylor will endeavor to take
advantage of the course to be given them at the Mayo
Clinic. They are serious minded and I am sure will
make diligent students.

     Again expressing the appreciation of the Sur-
geon General and the faculty of the Naval Medical
School, I am

                    Very sincerely,

                    Rear Admiral, Medical Corps, U.S.Navy.

THE ASHEVILLE CITIZEN

"DEDICATED TO THE UP-BUILDING OF WESTERN NORTH CAROLINA"

ESTABLISHED 1868.   ASHEVILLE, N. C., TUESDAY MORNING, MAY 29, 1923.   PRICE FIVE CENTS

ASHEVILLE, N. C., TUESDAY MORNING, MAY 29, 1923.

DR. C. S. NORBURN NAMED SURGEON TO THE PRESIDENT

Asheville Man Surgeon to Harding for the Alaskan Trip.

Dr. Charles S. Norburn, U.S.N., of this city. has been appointed surgeon to the President of the United States for the latter's Alaskan trip, and left Asheville yesterday afternoon for Washington, D. C., to sail aboard the transport "Henderson " from Norfolk, June 1.

The "Henderson," going to Alaska by way of the Panama Canal, will touch port on the Pacific Coast at San Francisco and there President Harding and the Presidential party, having gone across the continent by rail in order to meet the transport at this point will go abroad. From San Francisco the party will proceed to Alaska.

The nomination of Dr. Norburn for this important post was made by the surgeon-general of the navy, to whom Dr. Norburn's work is well known, and under whom Dr. Norburn worked when Dr. Stitt was an Admiral in the navy and since his present positions as surgeon-general. That so great an honor has come to an Asheville man has been the cause of much gratification locally, and also to the large circle of friends of Dr. Norburn's in the South And East.

Dr. Norburn is the son of Mr. and Mrs. Charles A. Norburn, to whom he has been paying a brief visit prior to leaving for his trip to Alaska. Dr. Norburn's rise to prominence in the navy started in 1917, when he volunteered for service at the outbreak of the World War. He was graduated a few weeks ahead of time from the University of Virginia in order to enter the United States Navy and left immediately after his graduation for Philadelphia where he took a course in general surgery at Dr. DaCosta's clinics Following this Dr. Norburn served upon the "Connecticut," the flagship of the Atlantic fleet, but did his greatest share of war work aboard the hospital ship. "Comfort, where his surgery first attracted particular attention. Series Of Honors Conferred Upon him.

The "Comfort" was used to transport the wounded from France and it was on board this vessel that Dr. Norburn's services as a surgeon covered a wide field.
LES BASSO

Scanned article from collection of Lillian N Alexander

The Norburn Hospital & Clinic

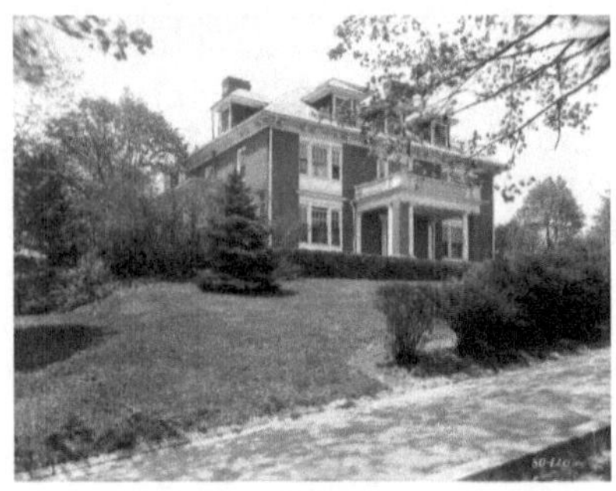

346 Montford Avenue, Asheville, NC
1928-1946

E. M. Ball, "Norburn Hospital," Photograph. Ramsey Library @ UNC Asheville/ Special Collections, n.d., accessed Oct. 10, 2021, http://toto.lib.unca.edu/findingaids/photo/ball/jpeg/ ball1317.jpg

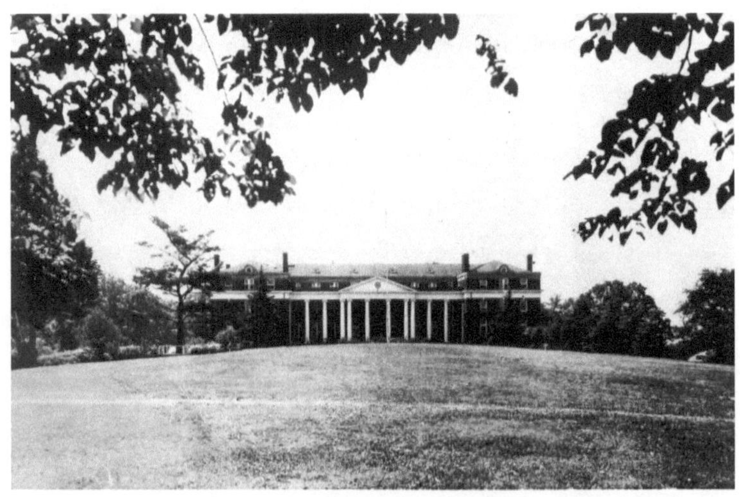

509 Biltmore Avenue, Asheville, NC
1946-1950

Photo courtesy of Joel Ingram of the Norburn family.

The Norburn Hospital & Clinic Medical Library

Excerpt from article "History of Buncombe County Medical Library," by Edgar Ward, October 8, 2017

In 1951 the merger of Memorial Mission Hospital and Victoria Hospital (previously the Norburn Hospital) enabled the society to move the library to a small brick building on the hospital grounds. The building already housed the Norburn Hospital Medical Library, which consisted primarily of the large and valuable medical library formerly belonging to Dr. Charles L. Norburn. Memorial Mission Hospital donated the Norburn Hospital Medical Library to the Library of the Buncombe County Medical Society.

The Norburn collection was an especially valuable addition. Among other items the library contained bound sets of medical journals, complete from the first issue, including forty-three volumes of the American Journal of Surgery, sixty-seven volumes of Surgery, Gynecology, and Obstetrics, one hundred eight volumes of the Annals of Surgery, and thirty-six volumes of the Archives of Surgery. . . .

The Library of the Buncombe County Medical Society lives on as the MAHEC Health Science Library . . . is linked by computer network to major libraries throughout the country. The staff includes a full-time director and four librarians. It is a major asset of the Memorial Mission-St. Joseph's Medical System and serves the needs of the sixteen western North Carolina counties.[10]

---

10. Silo.Tips, accessed June 16, 2021, https://silo.tips/download/
history-of-the-buncombe-county-medical-society

The Norburn Hospital & Clinic
Medical Librarian

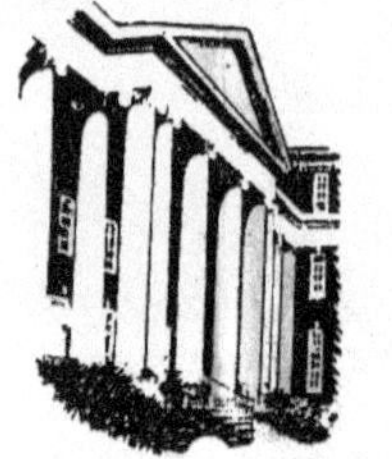

Dr. Charles S. Norburn
Valley Springs Road
Biltmore Forest,N.C.

Dear Dr. Charles:

It is with sincere regret that I learn you will no longer be
with the Hospital.

My year here as Librarian has been one of real happiness and
I want you to know that I have never worked anywhere that so
much interest and respect has been shown me and my work. It
is impossible for me to put into words my deep appreciation
for all your kindness.

Your years of serving humanity have been, I feel sure, hard
ones, but the comfort you have brought, the easing of pain and
the many lives you have saved will always live in the minds of
those you served: the good you have done and the ground-work
laid for this fine institution can never be extinguished.

Thanking you again for the frindship you have so generously
shown me and with all good wishes for the future, I remain,

Most sincerely,

Hattie E. McKay, Librarian

Letter from collection of Lillian N Alexander

EDITORIAL PAGE

THE ASHEVILLE TIMES

TUESDAY, DECEMBER 26, 1950

● Letters From Readers

ASHEVILLE'S FINE MEDICAL LIBRARY

EDITOR of The Times:
Asheville, N. C.

Your editorial in The Times, December 21, titled "New Medical Center Plan A Splendid Achievement" brought out the advantages of the amalgamation of the Victoria Hospital (formerly Norburn Hospital) and Memorial Mission Hospital.

One of these distinct advantages you mentioned was the Medical Library.

As I have had the privilege of being Medical Librarian for fourteen months at the Victoria Hospital (formerly Norburn Hospital) I know you, the medical profession and citizens of this section will be keenly interested in some pertinent facts regarding this particular library.

Dr. Charles S. Norburn, surgeon of renown, began his collection of these medical books and journals over thirty years ago. He spent much time and effort and spared no expense in securing the surgical journals he knew were a vital part of his work and library. At one time Dr. Norburn bought fifty volumes in order to secure two he needed to complete a file. One of the files dates back to 1885 and runs to date. Others which were edited at a later date are complete and his collection is one that is most outstanding as there are very few complete files throughout the country.

Of course this library has many books, some of which cannot be replaced. The total number of volumes, including bound journals, is well over three thousand. This library has meant much to the doctors and all departments of the hospital in solving difficult or unusual problems pertaining to their particular needs.

For one man to have built up such an amazing and valuable collection of journals and books, as Dr. Charles Norburn did, is something the people of these mountains may well be proud of and Memorial Mission Hospital has indeed inherited a rare jewel.

(MISS) HATTIE E. M'KAY
Medical Librarian
Victoria Hospital.

Dec. 23, 1950.
Asheville, N. C.

Letter from collection of Lillian N Alexander